PRACTICAL PERIODONTAL PLASTIC SURGERY

PRACTICAL PERIODONTAL PLASTIC SURGERY

Authors:

Serge Dibart, DMD
Associate Professor
Clinical Director Department of Periodontology and Oral Biology
Boston University School of Dental Medicine
100 East Newton Street
Boston, MA 02118

Mamdouh Karima, BDS, CAGS, DSc
Assistant Professor of Periodontics
Clinical Director
Faculty of Dentistry
King Abdulaziz University
PO Box 80209
Jeddah 21589, Saudi Arabia

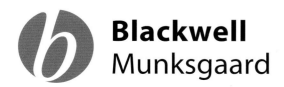

Blackwell
Munksgaard

Serge Dibart is clinical director of the periodontal residency program at Boston University Goldman School of Graduate Dentistry.

Mamdouh Karima is director of the periodontal residency program at King Abdulaziz University School of Dental Medicine in Saudi Arabia.

© 2006 by Serge Dibart and Mamdouh M. Karima, a Blackwell Publishing Company

Editorial Offices:
Blackwell Publishing Professional,
2121 State Avenue, Ames, Iowa 50014-8300, USA
    Tel: _1 515 292 0140
9600 Garsington Road, Oxford OX4 2DQ
    Tel: 01865 776868
Blackwell Publishing Asia Pty Ltd,
550 Swanston Street, Carlton South,
Victoria 3053, Australia
    Tel: _61 (0)3 9347 0300
Blackwell Wissenschafts Verlag, Kurfürstendamm 57,
10707 Berlin, Germany
    Tel: _49 (0)30 32 79 060

Europe and Asia

North America

Library of Congress
Cataloging-in-Publication Data
Dibart, Serge.
  Practical periodontal plastic surgery /
authors, Serge Dibart, Mamdouh
  Karima.—1st ed.
      p. ; cm.
  Includes bibliographical references.
  ISBN-13: 978-0-8138-2268-6 (alk. paper)
  ISBN-10: 0-8138-2268-8 (alk. paper)
  1. Periodontium—Surgery. 2. Surgery,
Plastic. I. Karima, Mamdouh.
  II. Title.
      [DNLM: 1. Periodontium—surgery.
2. Oral Surgical Procedures,
  Preprosthetic—methods. 3. Periodontics—methods.
    4. Reconstructive
  Surgical Procedures—methods.   WU 240
D543p 2006]
  RK361.D53 2006
  617.6*32059—dc22

2006001942

Set in Helvetica
by Dedicated Business Services
Printed and bound by COS

For further information on
Blackwell Publishing, visit our Dentistry Subject Site:
www.dentistry.blackwellmunksgaard.com

The last digit is the print number: 9 8 7 6 5 4 3 2

Contents

Contributors

James Belcher, DDS
Private practice limited to periodontics
3003 South Florida Avenue
Lakeland, FL 33803, USA
Telephone: (863) 687-9227
Fax: (863) 687-2813
E-mail: Belcher@lakelandperio.com
Founder and head of the Periodontal Microsurgical
    Institute, Lakeland, FL, USA

Diego Capri, DDS
Private practice limited to periodontics and dental implants
Via Loderingo degli Andolo
40124 Bologna, Italy
Telephone: 051-3399312
Fax: 051-332165
E-mail: Capri@fastwebnet.it

Serge Dibart, DMD
Associate Professor
Clinical Director
Department of Periodontology and Oral Biology
Boston University School of Dental Medicine
100 East Newton Street
Boston, MA 02118, USA
Telephone: (617) 638-4762
Fax: (617) 638-6170
E-mail: sdibart@bu.edu

Ming Fang Su, DMD, MSc
Assistant Clinical Professor
Department of Periodontology and Oral Biology
Boston University School of Dental Medicine
100 East Newton Street
Boston, MA 02118, USA
Telephone: (617) 638-4760
Fax: (617) 638-6170
E-mail: suming@bu.edu

Spencer N. Frankl, DDS, MSD, FICD, FACD
Professor and Dean
Boston University School of Dental Medicine
100 East Newton Street
Boston, MA 02118, USA

Mamdouh Karima, BDS, CAGS, DSc
Assistant Professor of Periodontics
Clinical Director
Faculty of Dentistry
King Abdulaziz University
PO Box 80209
Jeddah 21589, Saudi Arabia
Tel:(966)26401000 ext. 20030/20345
Fax (966)26403316
E-mail: mamdouhk_2000@yahoo.com

Luigi Montesani, MD, DMD
Private practice limited to periodontics, dental implants,
    and prosthodontics
Via Lazio 6
00187 Rome, Italy
Telephone: 06-4821722
Fax: 06-4823803
E-mail: luigi@montesani.it

Yu-Chuan Pan, MD
Microsurgery Course Director
Department of Plastic Surgery
University of Texas M.D. Anderson Cancer Center
1515 Holcombe Boulevard, Unit 443
Houston, TX 77030-4095, USA
Telephone: (713) 794-4030
Fax: (713) 794-5492
E-mail: ypan@mdanderson.org

Foreword

Readers of this book will gain invaluable, practical knowledge about periodontal surgery. Practitioners and students alike will learn the most up-to-date information they need to succeed in an increasingly technology-driven world.

As providers of patient care, we constantly need to be aware of improvements in our field—and how these improvements impact other specialties. By gaining a solid understanding of modern periodontal surgery, practitioners will be poised to take their practice to the next level, offering patients the best evidence-based procedures to improve their oral health.

There is nothing constant but change itself. With this in mind, Serge Dibart and Mamdouh Karima have focused not only on traditional periodontal interventions but also on the expanding field of periodontal microsurgery and increasingly popular aesthetic procedures along with other mucogingival operations. With their clear prose and expert, step-by-step instructions, they guide experienced practitioners and periodontal trainees alike in how to provide exceptional care for patients by using the newest, proven techniques.

After graduating from dental school, we have, in a sense, just begun our education. Here at Boston University, we use the "school without walls" model—where learning takes place both inside the four walls of the school and outside in our greater world community as well. Experienced periodontists know this to be the case: that learning continues after school and as traditional divisions are broken down among specialties. This book is one tool to update and reinforce your education and relevance in today's rapidly changing world.

Now, more than ever, oral health practitioners need to keep abreast of developments and scientific discoveries. This textbook expands the possibilities for learning and teaching.

Spencer N. Frankl, DDS, MSD, FICD, FACD
Professor and Dean
Boston University School of Dental Medicine

Acknowledgments

I thank my family for their financial and emotional support while on my journey to become a periodontist, especially my father, the late Dr. Henri Dibart, and my uncle, the late Dr. Nicolas Minassian.

I offer special thanks to my lifelong mentor, Dr. Paul Kaplanski, an outstanding practitioner and human being.

I extend all of my gratitude to Dean Spencer Frankl, without whom none of this would have been possible. He has been a beacon of light in my life (and others).

It is my pleasure to acknowledge the following colleagues, as well as the students and faculty of Boston University School of Dental Medicine, for their contribution to this book's manuscript: Ms. Leila Joy Rosenthal for illustrating Figures 2.1–2.5, 5.3, and 5.13; Dr. James Belcher for Figures 4.1–4.11; Dr. Luigi Montesani for Figures 5.9 and 5.14–5.17; Professor Alberto Barlattani for Figure 12.20; Dr. Haneen Bokhadoor for Figures 6.1, 6.3–6.5, and 12.31–12.35; Drs. Haneen Bokhadour and Nawaf Al-Dousari for Figures 15.15–15.23; Dr. Giacomo Ori for Figures 15.1, 15.2, and 15.12–15.14; Dr. Iain Chapple for Figures 15.3 and 15.4; Dr. Kemal Kose for Figures 7.1–7.4; Dr. Diego Capri for Figures 8.1–8.5 and 13.1–13.3; Dr. Ronaldo Santana for Figures 8.6–8.9; Dr. Takanari Myamoto for Figures 8.10–8.14 and 10.1–10.6; Dr. Hung Hui Chi for Figures 9.1–9.7, 11.4–11.8, and 12.1–12.10; Dr. Joseph Leary for Figures 10.7–10.10; Dr. Dina Macki for Figures 12.30, 12.38, and 12.39; Dr. Bassam Al Jamous for Figures 12.36 and 12.37; Dr. Albert Price for Figures 12.40–12.49 and 12.51; Dr. R. Deregis for Figure 12.50; Dr. Ekkasak Sornkul for Figures 15.7 and 15.11; Dr. Myra Brennan for Figure 14.13; Dr. Gianfranco Di Febo (prosthodontist) and Mr. Roberto Bonfiglioli (dental technician) for Figures 14.4, 14.16, and 14.70; Dr. Alessandro Cantagalli (prosthodontist) and Mr. Roberto Bonfiglioli (dental technician) for Figure 14.21; Dr. Alessandro Cantagalli (prosthodontist) and Mr. Giuseppe Mignani (dental technician) for Figure 14.24; Dr. Alessandro Cantagalli (prosthodontist) and Mr. Roberto Reggiani and Mr. Roberto Rivani (dental technicians) for Figures 14.26 and 14.28; Dr. Alessandro Cantagalli (prosthodontist) and Mr. Andrea Tondini (dental technician) for Figures 14.31 and 14.64; Dr. Massimo Fuzzi (prosthodontist) and Mr. Roberto Bonfiglioli (dental technician) for Figures 14.43 and 14.78; and Dr. Andrea Placci (prosthodontist) and Mr. Giuseppe Bonadia (dental technician) for Figure 14.87.

Last, but not least, I thank Ms. Jennifer DeSantis for helping with the preparation of the book's manuscript and Ms. Sophia Joyce, commissioning editor, for accepting to publish it.

Serge Dibart, DMD

Introduction

Mamdouh Karima

Mucogingival therapy is a general term describing nonsurgical and surgical treatment procedures for the correction of defects in morphology, position, and/or amount of soft tissue and underlying bony support around teeth and dental implants. The term *mucogingival surgery* was introduced in the literature by Friedman in 1957 and was defined as "surgical procedures for the correction of relationship between the gingiva and the oral mucous membrane with reference to problems associated with attached gingiva, shallow vestibules, and a frenum attachment that interfere with the marginal gingiva." Frequently, however, the term mucogingival surgery described all surgical procedures that involved both the gingiva and the alveolar mucosa.

Consequently, not only were techniques designed (a) to enhance the width of the gingiva and (b) to correct particular soft tissue defects regarded as mucogingival procedures, but included in this group of periodontal treatment modalities were (c) certain pocket-elimination approaches.

According to the latest version of the American Academy of Periodontology's *Glossary of Periodontal Terms* (1992), mucogingival surgery is defined as "plastic surgical procedures designed to correct defects in the morphology, position and/or amount of gingiva surrounding the teeth." Miller (1993) proposed that the term *periodontal plastic surgery* is more appropriate because mucogingival surgery has moved beyond the traditional treatment of problems associated with the amount of gingiva and recession-type defects to include correction of ridge form and soft tissue aesthetics. Consequently, periodontal plastic surgery is defined as "surgical procedures performed to prevent or correct anatomic, developmental, traumatic, or plaque disease-induced defects of the gingiva, alveolar mucosa, or bone" (American Academy of Periodontology 1996, p. 702).

REFERENCES

American Academy of Periodontology (1992) *Glossary of Periodontal Terms,* 3rd edition. Chicago: American Academy of Periodontology, 47.

American Academy of Periodontology (1996) Consensus report on mucogingival therapy. *Annals of Periodontology* 1, 701–706.

Friedman, N. (1957) Mucogingival surgery. *Texas Dental Journal* 75, 358–362.

Miller, P.D. (1993) Periodontal plastic surgery. *Current Opinion in Periodontology,* 136–143.

PRACTICAL PERIODONTAL PLASTIC SURGERY

Chapter 1: Definition and Objectives of Periodontal Plastic Surgery

Serge Dibart and Mamdouh Karima

Periodontal plastic surgery procedures are performed to prevent or correct anatomical, developmental, traumatic, or plaque disease–induced defects of the gingiva, alveolar mucosa, and bone [American Academy of Periodontology (AAP) 1996].

THERAPEUTIC SUCCESS

This is the establishment of a pleasing appearance and form for all periodontal plastic procedures.

INDICATIONS

Gingival augmentation

This is used to stop marginal tissue recession or to correct an alveolar bone dehiscence resulting from natural or orthodontically induced tooth movement. It facilitates plaque control around teeth or dental implants, or is used in conjunction with the placement of fixed partial dentures (Nevins 1986; Jemt et al. 1994).

Root coverage

The migration of the gingival margin below the cemento-enamel junction with exposure of the root surface is called *gingival recession*, which can affect all teeth surfaces, although it is most commonly found at the buccal surfaces. Gingival recession has been associated with tooth-brushing trauma, periodontal disease, tooth malposition, alveolar bone dehiscence, high muscle attachment, frenum pull, and iatrogenic dentistry (Wennstrom 1996). Gingival recessions can be classified in four categories based on the expected success rate for root coverage (Miller 1985):

- Class I: A recession not extending beyond the mucogingival line; normal interdental bone. Complete root coverage is expected.

- Class II: A recession extending beyond the mucogingival line; normal interdental bone. Complete root coverage is expected.

- Class III: A recession to or beyond the mucogingival line. There is a loss of interdental bone, with level coronal to gingival recession. Partial root coverage is expected.

- Class IV: A recession extending beyond the mucogingival line. There is a loss of interdental bone apical to the level of tissue recession. No root coverage is expected.

Root-coverage procedures are aimed at improving aesthetics, reducing root sensitivity, and managing root caries and abrasions.

Augmentation of the edentulous ridge

This is a correction of ridge deformities following tooth loss or developmental defects (Allen et al. 1985; Hawkins et al. 1991). It is used in preparation for the placement of a fixed partial denture or implant-supported prosthesis when aesthetics and function could be otherwise compromised. Ridge deformities can be grouped into three classes (Seibert 1993):

- Class I: A horizontal loss of tissue with normal, vertical ridge height

- Class II: Vertical loss of ridge height with normal, horizontal ridge width

- Class III: Combination of horizontal and vertical tissue loss

Aberrant frenulum

This is used to help close a diastema in conjunction with orthodontic therapy. It is used in treating gingival tissue recession aggravated by a frenum pull (Edwards 1977).

Prevention of ridge collapse associated with tooth extraction (socket preservation)

The maintenance of socket space with a bone graft after extraction will help reduce the chances of alveolar ridge resorption and facilitate future implant placement.

Crown Lengthening

This is used when there is not enough dental tissue available or to improve aesthetics (Bragger et al. 1992; Garber & Salama 1996).

Exposure of nonerupted teeth

The procedure is aimed at uncovering the clinical crown of a tooth that is impacted and enable its correct positioning on the arch through orthodontic movement.

Loss of interdental papilla

No technique can predictably restore a lost interdental papilla. The best way to restore a papilla is not to lose it in the first place.

FACTORS THAT AFFECT THE OUTCOME OF PERIODONTAL PLASTIC PROCEDURES

Teeth irregularity

Abnormal tooth alignment is a major cause of gingival deformities that require corrective surgery and is a significant factor in determining the outcomes of treatment. The location of the gingival margin, the width of the attached gingiva, and the alveolar bone height and thickness are all affected by tooth alignment.

On teeth that are tilted or rotated labially, the labial bony plate is thinner and located farther apically than on the adjacent teeth. The gingiva is receded, subsequently exposing the root. On the lingual surface of such teeth, the gingiva is bulbous and the bone margins are closer to the cemento-enamel junction. The level of gingival attachment on root surfaces and the width of the attached gingiva following mucogingival surgery are affected as much, or more, by tooth alignments as by variations in treatment procedures.

Orthodontic correction is indicated when performing mucogingival surgery on malpositioned teeth in an attempt to widen the attached gingiva or to restore the gingiva over denuded roots. If orthodontic treatment is not feasible, the prominent tooth should be ground to within the borders of the alveolar bone, avoiding pulp injury.

Roots covered with thin bony plates present a hazard in mucogingival surgery. Even the simplest type of flap (partial thickness) creates the risk of bone resorption on the periosteal surface (Hangorsky & Bissada 1980). Resorption in amounts that generally are not significant may cause loss of bone height when the bony plate is thin or tapered at the crest.

Mental nerve

The mental nerve emerges from the mental foramen, most commonly apical to the first and second mandibular premolars, and usually divides into three branches. One branch turns forward and downward to the skin of the chin. The other two branches travel forward and upward to supply the skin and mucous membrane of the lower lip and the mucosa of the labial alveolar surface.

Trauma to the mental nerve can produce uncomfortable paresthesia of the lower lip, from which recovery is slow. Familiarity with the location and appearance of the mental nerve reduces the likelihood of injuring it.

Muscle attachments

Tension from high muscle attachments interferes with mucogingival surgery by causing postoperative reduction in vestibular depth and width of the attached gingiva.

Mucogingival junction

Ordinarily, the mucogingival line in the incisor and canine area is located approximately 3 mm apically to the crest of the alveolar bone on the radicular surfaces and 5 mm interdentally (Strahan 1963). In periodontal disease and on malpositioned, disease-free teeth, the bone margin is located farther apically and may extend beyond the mucogingival line.

The distance between the mucogingival line and the cemento-enamel junction before and after periodontal surgery is not necessarily constant. After inflammation is eliminated, there is a tendency for the tissue to contract and draw the mucogingival line in the direction of the crown (Donnenfeld & Glickman 1966).

REFERENCES

Allen, E.P., Gainza, C.S., Farthing, G.G., & Newbold, D.A. (1985) Improved technique for localized ridge augmentation: A report of 21 cases. *Journal of Periodontology* 56, 195–199.

American Academy of Periodontology (AAP) (1996) Consensus report: Mucogingival therapy. *Annals of Periodontology* 1, 702–706.

Bragger, U., Lauchenauer, D., & Lang N.P. (1992) Surgical lengthening of the clinical crown. *Journal of Clinical Periodontology* 19, 58–63.

Donnenfeld, O.W., & Glickman, I. (1966) A biometric study of the effects of gingivectomy. *Journal of Periodontology* 36, 447–452.

Edwards, J.G. (1977) The diatema, the frenum, the frenectomy: A clinical study. *American Journal of Orthodontics* 71, 489–508.

Garber, D.A., & Salama, M.A. (1996) The aesthetic smile: Diagnosis and treatment. *Periodontology 2000* 11, 18–79.

Hangorsky, U., & Bissada, N.F. (1980) Clinical assessment of free gingival graft effectiveness on the maintenance of periodontal health. *Journal of Periodontology* 51, 274–278.

Hawkins, C.H., Sterrett, J.D., Murphy, H.J., & Thomas, R.C. (1991) Ridge contour related to esthetics and function. *Journal of Prosthetic Dentistry* 66, 165–168.

Jemt, T., Book, K., Lie, A., & Borjesson, T. (1994) Mucosal topography around implants in edentulous upper jaws: Photogrammetric three-dimensional measurements of the effect of replacement of a removable prosthesis with a fixed prosthesis. *Clinical Oral Implants Research* 5, 220–228.

Miller, P.D. (1985) A classification of marginal tissue recession. *International Journal of Periodontics and Restorative Dentistry* 5(2), 8–13.

Nevins, M. (1986) Attached gingival-mucogingival therapy and restorative dentistry. *International Journal of Periodontics and Restorative Dentistry* 6(4), 9–27.

Seibert, J.S. (1993) Reconstruction of the partially edentulous ridge: Gateway to improved prosthetics and superior aesthetics. *Practical Periodontics and Aesthetic Dentistry* 5, 47–55.

Strahan, J.D. (1963) The relation of the mucogingival junction to the alveolar bone margin. *Dental Practitioner and Dental Record* 14, 72–74.

Wennstrom, J.L. (1996) Mucogingival therapy. *Annals of Periodontology* 1, 671–701.

Chapter 2: Surgical Armamentarium, Sutures, Anesthesia, and Postoperative Management

Serge Dibart

ARMAMENTARIUM

This includes the basic surgical kit:

- Mouth mirror
- Periodontal probe (UNC15; Hu-Friedy, Chicago, IL, USA)
- College pliers (DP2; Hu-Friedy)
- Scalpel handle no. 5 (Hu-Friedy) with blade no. 15 or 15C
- Tissue pliers (TPKN; Hu-Friedy)
- Periosteal elevator 24G (Hu-Friedy)
- Prichard periosteal elevator (PR-3; Hu-Friedy)
- Gracey curette 11/12 or Younger-Good universal curette (Hu-Friedy)
- Rhodes back-action periodontal chisel (Hu-Friedy)
- Castroviejo needle holder (Hu-Friedy)
- Goldman-Fox curved scissors (Hu-Friedy)
- A 5-0 silk suture with P-3 needle
- A 5-0 chromic gut suture with C-3 needle
- Periodontal dressing

For basic microsurgical procedures, add the following to the kit:

- Magnifying loupes ×4 (or higher) wide field or surgical microscope
- Surgical headlight (optional)
- Miniblade scalpel handle with miniblades (round tip and spoon blade angle of 2.5 mm)
- Micro Castroviejo needle holder
- Castroviejo curved microsurgical scissors
- Microsurgical tissue pliers
- A 6-0 chromic gut suture with C-1 needle
- A 7-0 coated vicryl suture 3/8 with 6.6-mm needle

SUTURES

Use the smallest and least reactive suture material compatible with the surgical problem (Halstead 1913).

Types

Two major categories of suture materials exist—resorbable and nonresorbable. These sutures are best used with tapercut needles, which have a sharp point and pass atraumatically through the mucogingival tissue, making them ideal for periodontal plastic surgery use.

Nonresorbable sutures

Silk (braided)

A silk suture is easy to use, and its smooth handling ensures knot security. A disadvantage, however, is that it will absorb plaque and may infect the wound if kept longer than 1 week.

Polyester (nylon monofilament, polytetrafluoroethylene)

The polyester suture can be kept in the mouth longer, for 2–3 weeks, with little risk of infection. A disadvantage is that it is likely to untie if extreme care is not exerted when tying the knot. This is a result of the materials' characteristics.

Resorbable sutures

Gut

A gut suture has mild tensile strength and is resorbed by the body's enzymes in approximately 5–7 days. A disadvantage is that its knot-handling properties are inferior to those of silk sutures. Gut sutures may untie, so care must be taken not to cut the ends too short. Gut sutures may also irritate the tissues.

Chromic gut

A chromic gut suture has moderate tensile strength and is resorbed in 7–10 days. This suture is more practical than the gut suture.

Polyglycolic acid (synthetic)

The polyglycolic acid suture has good tensile strength, resorbs slowly (within 3–4 weeks intraorally), and is broken down through slow hydrolysis.

Sizes

Suture sizes vary from 1-0 to 10-0, with 10-0 being the thinnest. The most common size used for periodontal plastic macrosurgery is 5-0, and the most common sizes used for periodontal microsurgery are 6-0, 7-0, and 8-0.

Cyanoacrylates (butyl and isobutyl forms)

Cyanoacrylate sutures have been used in wound closure since the mid-1960s. The cyanoacrylates can cement tissues together and dissolve in 4–7 days (McGraw & Caffesse 1978). These sutures should not be used alone to secure wound closure, but can be used as an adjunct to sutures.

Techniques

- Single interrupted suture (Fig. 2.1)
- Horizontal mattress suture (Fig. 2.2)
- Vertical mattress suture (Fig. 2.3)
- Crisscross suture (Fig. 2.4)
- Sling suture (Fig. 2.5)

ANESTHESIA

Most of the time, adequate and profound anesthesia for soft tissue resection and limited bone contouring may be secured through infiltration. Block anesthesia may reduce the number of needle punctures in nonanesthetized tissue, but infiltration will achieve tissue rigidity and hemostasis that are useful when proceeding with the incisions.

Necessary armamentarium

- 10 ml Chlorhexidine gluconate 0.12
- Topical anesthetic and application tip
- Anesthetic aspirating syringe
- 30-Gauge needle
- Lidocaine hydrochloride (HCl) with 1/100,000 epinephrine
- Lidocaine HCl with 1/50,000 epinephrine (to control hemorrhaging only)

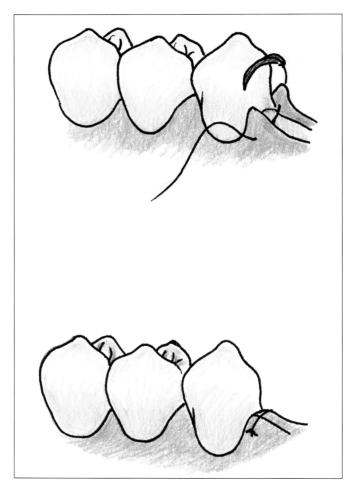

Figure 2.1. Single interrupted suture.

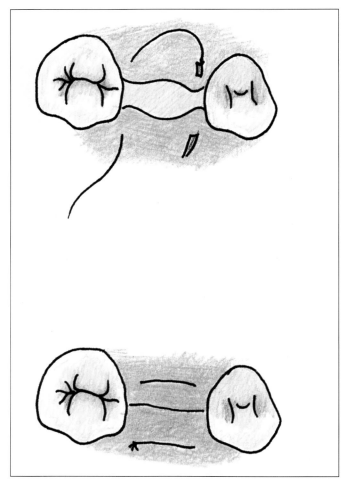

Figure 2.2. Horizontal mattress sutures.

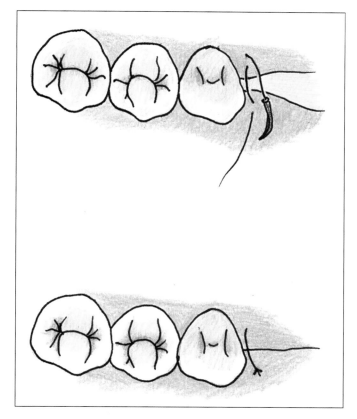

Figure 2.3. Vertical mattress suture.

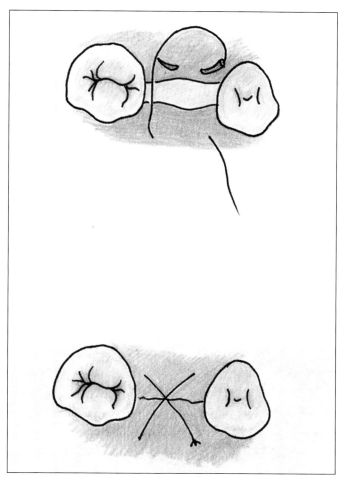

Figure 2.4. Crisscross suture.

Technique

After the patient rinses for 1 min with 10 ml of chlorhexidine gluconate, dry the areas to be anesthetized with a gauze. Using a Q-tip, apply the topical anesthetic on the oral tissues for 3 min for superficial anesthesia. Then anesthetize locally using one or two carpules of Lidocaine HCl with 1/100,000 epinephrine in infiltration. Distraction techniques, such as gently pressing the tissues at some distance of the intended puncture site, may help further diminish the perception of puncture pain.

The first step is to administer the injection to the vestibular fold and then inject small amounts of anesthetic into the interdental papillae of the surgical site (buccal and palatal/lingual). You will observe blanching of the papilla being anesthetized, the marginal gingiva, and the adjacent papilla. This will help provide a painless anesthesia as you move along the area to be anesthetized.

Diffuse the anesthetic by gently massaging the soft tissues of the vestibular fold with your finger. This will reduce the swelling occasioned by the anesthetic solution. At this time, you will be able to see your anatomical landmarks again. Massaging the tissue will also promote their rapid anesthesia.

A few drops of lidocaine HCl with 1/50,000 epinephrine can be used to control bleeding by infiltrating the tissues around the surgical site.

POSTOPERATIVE INSTRUCTIONS, MEDICATIONS, AND REGIMEN

After the procedure, the patient is given a mild analgesic while still in the office (i.e., ibuprofen 600 mg) as well as an ice pack.

Prescription

1. Ibuprofen 600 mg (Motrin) or acetaminophen 300 mg and codeine phosphate 30 mg (Tylenol no. 3) 3–4 times a day as needed for pain.

2. Chlorhexidine gluconate 0.12% to be used after week 1. Rinse twice a day for 7 days.

Instructions

Instruct the patient to keep the ice on the face for the next 2 h, 20 min on and 20 min off. Also instruct the patient to

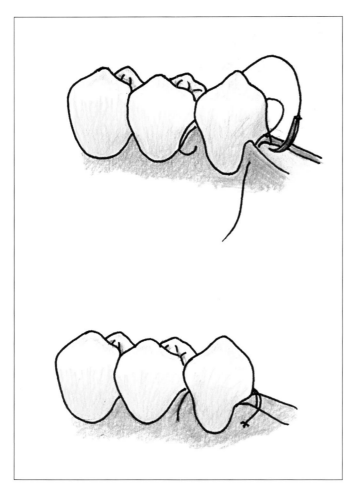

Figure 2.5. Sling suture.

Specific instructions after soft tissue grafting

Emphasize to the patient that the 4 days following the surgery are critical for the success of the graft. It should be remembered that, when transplanted, a diffusion system will maintain both the graft's epithelium and connective tissue for approximately 3 days until circulation is restored (Foman 1960); therefore, complete immobility of the graft is a must for a successful outcome of the procedure. After suture removal, the patient should not brush the grafted area for 2 weeks. Two weeks after surgery a Q-tip, dipped in chlorhexidine gluconate, should be used in lieu of a toothbrush to clean the teeth of the grafted site. The patient should continue this for 2 months. After a 2-month period, gentle brushing of the area can be initiated.

REFERENCES

Foman, S. (1960) *Cosmetic Surgery.* Philadelphia: Lippincott, 161–200.

Halstead, W.S. (1913) Ligature and suture material. *Journal of the American Medical Association* 60, 119–125.

McGraw, V., & Caffesse, R. (1978) Cyanoacrylates in periodontics. *Journal of the Western Society of Periodontology/Periodontal Abstracts* 26, 4–13.

keep a soft diet and to avoid alcoholic beverages and hot or spicy food for the next 48 h. The patient should also refrain from rinsing, physical exercise, and taking drugs containing aspirin.

The sutures, if nonresorbable, will be removed after 1 week, and the patient will be asked to rinse with chlorhexidine gluconate 1.2% for 1 week after the removal of the sutures.

Chapter 3: Introduction to Microsurgery and Training

Ming Fang Su and Yu-Chuan Pan

INTRODUCTION

In 1960, J.H. Jacobson and E.L. Suarez first introduced microsurgical technique when they anastomosed small vessels under an operative microscope. In 1963, Chen Zong-Wei, the authoritative figure in microsurgery in China, reported the world's first successful replantation of an amputated forearm (Chen et al 1963a & b). Thereafter, with the development and refinement of microsurgical technique and its clinical application, much progress has been made in reconstructive surgery throughout the world.

TRAINING IN MICROSURGERY

Generally speaking, microsurgery techniques are comparatively difficult to learn. Learning microsurgical skills requires practice that involves a period of hardship and endurance. Before the clinical application in patients, it is paramount that one train in the laboratory and on animal models to gain familiarity with techniques.

Since viewing objects under the microscope or surgical loupes is different from viewing objects with the naked eye, a surgeon's hand-eye coordination must be precisely adjusted according to various degrees of magnification. The hands must be trained for delicate manipulation. This is one of the challenges in microsurgery. The higher the magnification is, the more accurate the maneuvering that is required.

BASIC MICROINSTRUMENTATION

Few items are required for the training in microsurgery (Fig. 3.1).

Microsurgery basic set

The five pieces are:

- One curved, 14-m-long microneedle holder
- Two straight, 15-cm-long micro–strong forceps, with a 0.3-mm tip and round handle with platform
- One straight, 15-cm-long forceps, with a 0.2-mm tip and round handle with platform
- One straight, 14-cm-long scissors

Other surgical instruments and materials

These include:

- Straight, 12.5-cm-long Adson forceps (Microsurgery Instruments, Bellaire, TX, USA), with 1 × 2 teeth

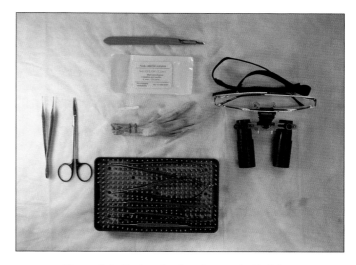

Figure 3.1. Basic setup for microsurgical training.

- Curved, 12.5-cm-long Iris scissors (Microsurgery Instruments)
- Suture card with 16 lines for suture practice
- Vascular double clamps
- Irrigating needle and spring

Microneedle holder

The needle holder is used to grasp the needle, pull it through the tissues, and tie knots. The needle should be held between its middle and lower thirds at its distal tip. If the needle is held too close to the top, the anastomosis between the two ends of the vessel cannot be completed with a single stitch. If it is held too close to the bottom, maintaining steady control is difficult, and the direction of the tip can be changed easily. The needle can be bent or broken if too much force is used.

The needle holder is mainly manipulated by the thumb, index, and middle fingers, similar to how a pencil is held between the fingers. With this pencil-holding posture, the hand is maintained in a functional or neutral position.

The appropriate needle-holder length depends on the nature of the operation. The most commonly used are 14 cm and 18 cm. The tips can be straight or gently curved, but the latter are most often used. The choice of the tip is determined by the nature of the suture. Usually a delicate tip (0.3 mm) is used for 8-0 and 10-0 sutures. The needle holder with a 1-mm tip is used for 5-0 and 6-0 sutures.

Dentists commonly use a locking-type needle holder. A locking needle holder is useful because one can hold the needle securely, which is most important during needle insertion. To minimize jogging, the lock should be closed slowly but released promptly. Dedicated practice is necessary to develop skillful manipulation of the needle holder.

A needle holder should ensure that a needle is held steadily without slipping. It should be light and require the minimal force from the hand. It should be a length to suit the size of the hand and be manipulated easily. A titanium needle holder is the best choice.

Microforceps

These are important instruments in microsurgery, especially for delicate manipulation and detailed movement. They are used to handle minute tissues without damaging them and to hold fine sutures while tying knots. Microforceps can make those maneuvers that cannot be performed by hand. For example, the forceps can be inserted into the lumen of a cut vessel end to open the vascular lumen for needle insertion. The forceps used for vessel anastomosis are very fine and called *dilators*.

A standard pair of forceps should be able to pick up a 10-0 nylon suture on a glass board without slipping. The tips of the forceps should be smooth and strong. The forceps should not damage the tissue, and no break to the suture should occur during suturing.

Microdissection

Microforceps are used for dissection, especially for blood vessels and nerves. A common mistake occurs when the tips of the forceps adhere to the vessel wall, and the vessel breaks, which leads to massive bleeding. Therefore, when using the forceps for dissection, the artery and the vein should not be touched with the tips, which should be kept closed. The sides of the tips are used for dissection of tissues and blood vessels, similar to how fingers are used during blunt dissection in general surgery.

To prevent unnecessary bleeding, it is important to remember to use the *sides* of the tips for dissection so that the tips do not face and break the vessels. Delicate dissection can be performed after one is familiar with the use of microforceps. Even 0.3- to 0.5-mm blood vessels or nerves can be handled after repeated practice.

There are different types of microforceps for different operations. The most commonly used microforceps are 15 cm long, with round handles and 0.2- to 0.3-mm tips. The rounded handle enables the direction, degree, and position of the instrument to be changed by merely rolling the fingers, which facilitates knotting and dissection. The tips for microforceps can be straight or curved. Some have teeth to strengthen the opposing force of the tips, and some also have platforms. When operating on deeper structures, like the posterior part of the oral cavity, 18-cm-long forceps are used for dissection and for tying knots.

Jeweler forceps are strong and cheap, with a variety of tips available. They can be straight or curved at different degrees, such as 45° or 90°. They are usually 11–12 cm long and suitable only for superficial operations. Their handles are flat, which makes rotating and changing the direction of the instrument less efficient.

While stitching with a needle holder and forceps, the needle sometimes isn't in the microscopic field of view. Two different methods are adopted to find the missing needle. The first is to place the needle within the operating field under the microscope after every stitch. This is not only the easiest method but also the most time efficient. In the other method, the forceps are used to grasp one end of the thread, which slides through the tips of the forceps. The needle holder can catch the thread while the needle is seen. This should be done under the microscope to reduce operating time.

Microscissors

These are used for the dissection of tissues, blood vessels, and nerves. Different sizes of scissors are used for cutting sutures or tissue, removing adventitial tissue of vessels or nerves, and trimming vessels or nerves during repair.

The most commonly used microscissors are 14 cm and 18 cm long. To manage the delicate part of the adventitial tissues, 9-cm microscissors are preferable.

The tips of the scissor blades can be straight or gently curved. Straight scissors cut sutures and trim the adventitia of vessels or nerve endings. Curved scissors dissect vessels and nerves. The tips of the scissors should be sharp and cut with ease. During dissection of tissues and vessels, apart from using the tips to cut, the sides of the scissors can be used for dissection with the tips closed, similar to dissection with forceps. If done properly, it is a safe and fast way to use the tips of the scissors for dissection.

Surgical loupes

Since the mid-1960s, surgical loupes have been widely applied in microsurgery. In addition to the conventional role in pedicle dissection and flap elevation, they are also used in digital replantation, free jejunal transfer, and animal experimentation (Peters et al. 1971; McManammy 1983; Jurkiewicz 1984; Lee 1985; Shenaq et al. 1995).

Because of the exponential growth of the development of surgical loupes, those with a magnification of 2.5- to 4-fold and 5.5- to 8-fold are available.

The advantages of surgical loupes are that they are small, easy to carry, efficient, and cost-effective. If operating on a blood vessel of 1-mm diameter or larger with surgical loupes, the result will be the same as when working under a microscope. The most commonly used magnifications are 3.5- to 6.5-fold. A disadvantage of loupes is the limited magnifying power.

There are generally two types of surgical loupes:

Galilean loupes

These, which are economical and simple to use, consist of 2–3 lenses and are easy to operate, light, and inexpensive. Their disadvantages are limited magnification (2.5- or 3.5-fold) and a blurry peripheral border of the visual field.

Prism loupes (or wide-field loupes)

Each of the prism loupes, which are high quality and precise, consists of seven lenses. The magnification can reach from 3.5-fold to 10-fold, and the visual field is much clearer and sharper than with other loupes.

Properties of ideal surgical loupes

These include:

- Light weight: No pressure is felt on the nose bridge while wearing these loupes

- Advanced optic lenses: These have a clearer image, wider field of view, sharper picture, and a greater depth of visual field

- Vertical and interpupillary adjustment: This enables the operation to be performed with a comfortable posture

- Magnification (range, 2.5- to 8-fold) and working distances (range, 14–22 inches)

- Mounting choice: Spectacle frames and headband

- Low cost

The usual magnification of loupes for a general dentist is 2.5- to 3.5-fold. However, the magnification for a periodontist is 3.5- to 4.5-fold. The operation on delicate tissues requires loupes with a magnification of 5.5- to 6.5-fold.

Practice

It is an important step in practice to choose a pair of surgical loupes of appropriate magnification and comfortable working distance.

Proper wear

While wearing surgical loupes, along with adjusting inter-pupillary and vertical distances, the band of the surgical loupes must be fixed with appropriate tightness. If the band is too tight, too much force will be exerted on the nose bridge and the head, which is uncomfortable. Pain over the nose and head, and even swelling of the soft tissue, can occur after prolonged operations if the band is too tight.

Once the band length has been appropriately adjusted, the loupes should be moved up and down 1 cm over the nose. Properly fitted loupes exert no pressure onto the nose.

Adjusting the interpupillary and vertical distances for head-mounted bend loupes is necessary. The closer the lenses are to the eyes, the larger is the field of view. A comfortable size of the bend is also mandatory.

Focus

Focus is the primary aim for using surgical loupes properly. If the loupes are in focus, a clear operating view is obtained, facilitating the procedure. The focus is achieved by moving the head forward and backward until the head position can be maintained.

To obtain the proper focus, repeated exercises in head and neck positioning are needed. A simple way of doing this is to use a pair of surgical loupes to read newspapers or books. After practicing this 20–30 times every day for 3–5 days, it is easier to use loupes during microsurgery. To keep the loupes in focus during reading, the muscles of the head and the neck must be trained to maintain the head position. Once this is achieved, surgical loupes can be efficiently used during operations.

SUTURING TECHNIQUES

For suturing in microsurgery, microsutures from 8-0 to 11-0 are used. The largest sutures used in current microsurgical techniques, 8-0 sutures, are often chosen for use by novices; 9-0 sutures are used for 1- to 2-mm-vessel anastomosis; 10-0 sutures are used to repair small arteries or veins with a nerve diameter of less than 1 mm; and 11-0 sutures, the least commonly used, are reserved for special situations.

Suture card

This device used to practice suturing is made of silicon rubber or plastic and divided into 16 squares. Incisions are made on the silicon sheet in each square. A total of 16 suture lines are incised at four different directions, and 20–24 stitches are required to complete each suture line.

A total of more than 350 stitches can be made in each suture card. Different sized sutures can be practiced on this card to refine technique (Fig. 3.2).

The number of stitches made on a single suture card is equivalent to 1 year of experience of a surgeon practicing microsurgery. The reasoning behind this, for example, is that in a general hospital a plastic surgeon handles two cases of microsurgery each month and two anastomoses for each case, one for artery and one for vein. Four anastomoses are then made during each month, and each anastomosis takes eight stitches. In 1 month, 32 stitches are made and, in 1 year, 384 stitches are sutured. That is equivalent to the total on a single suture card.

Quality stitching

There is much emphasis not only on the quantity of the sutures, but also the quality. A quality stitch is required for each suture. Several requirements must be fulfilled when a stitch is made. First, stitches should be exactly 90° to the incisions. Second, every stitch should be the same size. If the size of the stitches differs, smoothness of the interior surface of the vessel cannot be maintained. This results in clot formation and leads to thrombosis. Third, the entry site and the exit site of every stitch should be the same width. Finally, the stitches should be equally spaced. Leaking may occur if the spacing of the stitches is uneven.

AN ANIMAL MODEL FOR MICROSURGERY TECHNIQUE TRAINING

During the training for microsurgery, every trainee has to learn the technique for tying, transplanting, and repairing different vessels, nerves, and tissue. Beginners have to practice on experimental animals to acquire the skill. The chicken leg is an effective and useful microsurgical teaching model (Fig. 3.3).

A chicken leg is a composite tissue with skin, fascia, muscle, nerve, artery, vein, and bone. It is a convenient and useful practicing material for a beginner in microsurgery, and is also readily available in supermarkets. To begin, the chicken leg is fixed on a wooden board with tape. The skin at the back is cut open to expose the fascia, muscles, nerves, and vessels. The artery length is 2–2.5 cm, with a diameter of 1.5 mm. Anastomosis can be performed up to three times on an artery. The diameter of a vein is 2–3 mm.

The openings for the artery and the vein are located at the back of the knee joint. They are both underneath the fascia and at the edge of the muscle, which can be observed with ease using surgical loupes or a microscope. The tissue is vertically dissected underneath the fascia with a pair of scissors to expose the artery, which is a pink figure beside the nerve. This blood vessel is suitable for practicing anastomosis, familiarizing oneself with the operation of a microscope or surgical loupes with 5.5- to 6.5-fold magnification, and coordinating hand-eye movements. Dye may be injected into an anastomosed vessel to assess the patency and observe any leakage. Training may continue on the chicken's fascial tissue, nerve, vein, and bone.

Once 30–50 anastomoses have been completed, one's skills and technique have greatly improved.

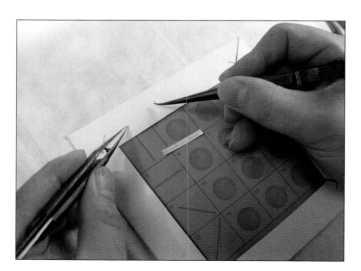

Figure 3.2. Microsurgical suturing exercise.

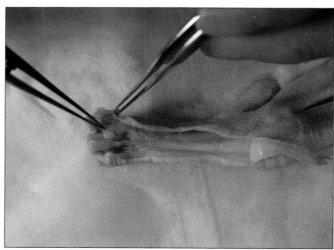

Figure 3.3. Dissection of a chicken foot, exposing an artery, a tendon, and a vein.

REFERENCES

Chen, Z.-W., et al. (1963a) Replantation of an amputated forearm. *Chinese Journal of Surgery* 11, 767.

Chen, Z.-W., Chen, Y.C., & Pao, Y.S. (1963b) Salvage of the forearm following complete amputation: Report of a case. *Chinese Medical Journal* 82, 632.

Jacobson, J.H., & Suarez, E.L. (1960) Microsurgery in anastomosis of small vessels [Abstract]. *Surgical Forum* 11, 243–245.

Jurkiewicz, M.J. (1984) Reconstructive surgery of the cervical esophagus. *Journal of Thoracic Surgery* 88, 893–897.

Lee, S. (1985) Historical Review of Microsurgery. In: Lee, S., ed. *Manual of Microsurgery*. Boca Raton, FL: CRC, 1–3.

McManammy, D.S. (1983) Comparison of microscope and loupe magnification: Assistance for the repair of median and ulnar nerves. *British Journal of Plastic Surgery* 36, 367–372.

Peters, C.R., McKee, D.M., & Berry, B.E. (1971) Pharyngoesophageal reconstruction with revascularized jejunal transplants. *American Journal of Surgery* 121, 675–678.

Shenaq, S.M., Klebuc, M.J.A., & Vargo, D. (1995) Free-tissue transfer with the aid of loupe magnification: Experience with 251 procedures. *Plastic and Reconstructive Surgery* 95, 261–269.

Chapter 4: Periodontal Microsurgery

James Belcher

HISTORICAL PERSPECTIVE

References to magnification date back 2,800 years, when simple glass meniscus lenses were described in ancient Egyptian writings. In 1694, Amsterdam merchant Anton van Leeuwenhook constructed the first compound-lens microscope. Magnification for microsurgical procedures was introduced to medicine during the late 1800s. In 1921, Carl Nylen, who is considered the father of microsurgery, first used the binocular microscope for ear surgery (Dohlman 1969). It was not until 1960, when Jacobsen and Suarez obtained 100% patency in suturing 1-mm-diameter blood vessels for anastomosis, that the surgical microscope gained wide acceptance in medicine (Barraquer 1980).

Apotheker & Jako (1981) first introduced the microscope to dentistry in 1978. During 1992, Carr published an article outlining the use of the surgical microscope during endodontic procedures. In 1993, Shanelec & Tibbetts (1998) presented a continuing-education course on periodontal microsurgery at the annual meeting of the American Academy of Periodontology. This led to centers devoted to teaching periodontists and other dentists periodontal microsurgery.

Belcher wrote an article in 2001 summarizing the benefits and potential usages of the surgical microscope in periodontal therapy. Although Belcher and several other periodontists view the addition of the microscope as an invaluable tool in periodontal therapy, it has been cautiously accepted by the periodontal profession as a whole.

PERIODONTAL APPLICATIONS

The operating microscope offers three distinct advantages to periodontists: illumination, magnification, and increased precision of surgical skills (Belcher 2001). The synergy of improved illumination and increased visual acuity enables the increased precision of surgical skills. Collectively, these advantages can be referred to as the *microsurgical triad* (Fig. 4.1).

Among many basic surgical principles, several are germane to periodontal surgery. Eliminating dead space, tissue handling, removal of necrotic tissue and foreign materials, closure with sufficient but appropriate tension, and immobilization of the wound are important surgical goals in periodontal therapy (Johnson & Johnson 1994, p. 9). The surgical operating microscope and appropriate microsurgical technique afford surgeons a more realistic chance of achieving these goals.

In periodontics, the surgical operating microscope, though useful in most areas of periodontal therapy, is particularly useful in mucogingival surgery, root preparation, and crown-lengthening procedures.

Microsurgical techniques are especially beneficial to mucogingival procedures. As mentioned, principles of wound healing require minimal dead space. The microscope enables clinicians to use smaller needles, sutures, and instruments, and precisely position tissues and stabilize the mending tissues.

Root preparation is an important modality in periodontal therapy. Lindhe & Nyman (1984) have suggested the success of periodontal therapy is due to the thoroughness of debridement of the root surface. Data show that surgical access improves the ability to remove calculus (Cobb 1996). Furthermore, research demonstrates that root preparation is enhanced when performed under illumination (Reinhardt et al. 1985). The surgical microscope provides fiber optic lighting and magnification for calculus removal.

Most published articles embracing the benefits of magnification in dentistry have been anecdotal (Campbell 1989). However, two articles do show enhanced clinical benefits of magnification. Leknius & Geissberger (1995) have shown a direct relationship between magnification and significantly enhanced performance of prosthodontic dental procedures.

A recently published article concluded that performing root-coverage techniques microsurgically versus macrosurgically substantially improved the vascularization of

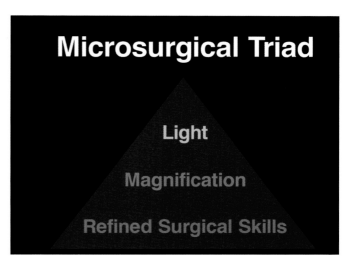

Figure 4.1. Microsurgical triad.

connective tissue grafts and the percentage of additional root coverage (Burdhardt & Lang 2005). There is a lack of studies in dentistry comparing the benefits of crown lengthening or other surgical procedures via standard versus microsurgical methods. Yet, it seems logical that if magnification is beneficial in prosthetics and root coverage, the surgical microscope, with its magnification, would aid practitioners in crown lengthening, root preparation, and other periodontal surgical procedures.

PERIODONTAL INSTRUMENTATION

Magnification enables dentists to use smaller instrumentation with more precision. Although the variety of microsurgical instrumentation designed for periodontal therapy is vast, the instrumentation can be divided into the following subgroups: knives, retractors, scissors, needle holders, tying forceps, and others.

The knives most commonly used in periodontal microsurgery are those used in ophthalmic surgery: blade breaker, crescent, minicrescent, spoon, lamella, and scleral knives (Fig. 4.2). Common characteristics of these knives are their extreme sharpness and small size. This enables precise incisions and maneuvers in small areas (Fig. 4.3).

The blade-breaker knife has a handle onto which a piece of an ophthalmic razor blade is affixed. This allows for infinite angulations of the blade. This knife is often used in place of a no. 15 blade.

The crescent knife can be used for intrasulcular procedures. It is available with one-piece handles or as a removable blade. It can be used in connective tissue graft proce-

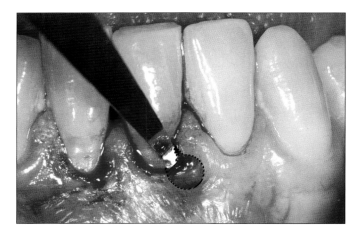

Figure 4.3. Spoon knife shown in sulcular undermining incision.

dures to obtain the donor graft, to tunnel under tissue, and to prepare the recipient site.

The spoon knife is beveled on one side, allowing the knife to track through the tissue adjacent to bone. It is frequently used in microsurgical procedures to undermine tissue, enhancing the placement of a connective tissue graft.

Retractors and elevators have been downsized. Scissors such as the micro–vannas tissue scissors are used for removal of small fragments of tissue. Needle holders are also downsized from sizes designed for conventional periodontal surgery. Tying forceps are an essential component of two-hand microsurgical tying. They are available in two general styles: platform and nonplatform. Several designs of both needle holders and tying forceps are available.

Microsurgical instrumentation can be made with titanium or surgical stainless steel. Titanium instruments tend to be lighter, but are more prone to deformation and are usually more expensive. Stainless-steel instruments are prone to magnetization, but there is a greater number and wider variety of them.

Needles and sutures

As mentioned earlier, basic surgical techniques are used to eliminate dead space, close a wound with sufficient but appropriate tension, and immobilize a wound (Johnson & Johnson 1994, p. 9). The appropriate combination of a properly selected needle and suture greatly contributes to the success of these techniques.

The most common curvature of needles used in dentistry is three-eighths inch (10 mm) and one-half inch (12.7 mm), the former being the most common (Fig. 4.4a). Dentists frequently use larger needles, such as 16–19 mm. Although larger needles are appropriate in certain surgical proce-

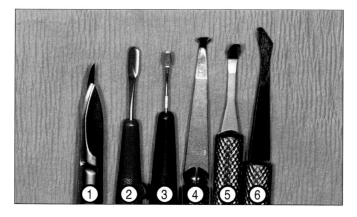

Figure 4.2. Periodontal microsurgical knives: *1*, blade breaker; *2*, crescent; *3*, minicrescent; *4*, 260° spoon; *5*, lamella, and *6*, sclera.

dures, such as flap closure after extractions, smaller needles enable precise closure of the mending tissues in more detailed procedures.

A spatula needle, which is beneficial in periodontal microsurgical procedures, is 6.6 mm long and has a curvature of 140° (Fig. 4.4b). The combination of a shallow needle tract and precise needle purchase of the tissue enables extremely accurate apposition and closure in periodontal mucogingival surgery.

An accepted surgical practice is to use the smallest suture possible to hold the mending tissue adequately (Johnson & Johnson 1994, p. 15). This practice minimizes the opening made by the needle and the trauma through the tissues. Frequently in periodontal microsurgical procedures, 6-0, 7-0, and 8-0 sutures are indicated.

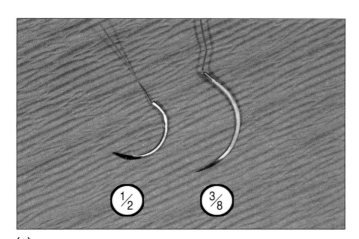

(a)

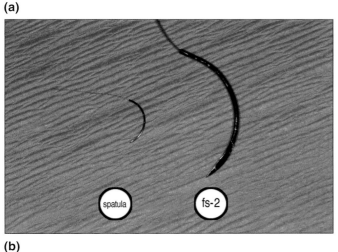

(b)

Figure 4.4. a: One-half-inch and three-eighths-inch curved needles. **b:** Spatula needle (6.6 mm) compared to FS-2 needle (19 mm).

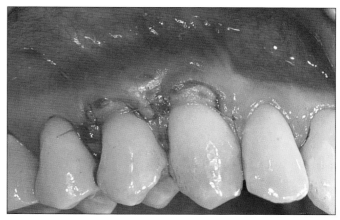

(a)

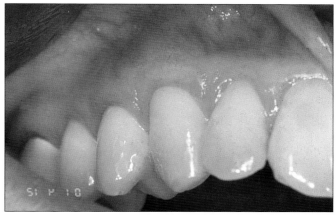

(b)

Figure 4.5. a: Connective tissue graft (CTG) placement via tunnel technique. **b:** Final healing of CTG.

Sutures can be classified as nonresorbable and resorbable, and can be multifilament or monofilament in design. Examples of nonresorbable sutures are silk, nylon, and polyester. Common resorbable sutures are plain and chromic gut, polyglactin 910, poliglecaprone 25, and polydioxanone. Medical studies have shown the superiority of poliglecaprone 25 and polyglactin 910 to gut (LaBabnara 1995; Anatol et al. 1997).

The combination of using smaller needles, sutures, and magnification results in minimal dead space, closure with sufficient but appropriate tension, and immobilization of the wound (Fig. 4.5).

Microsurgical tying

Several principles of microsurgical tying are applicable to periodontal therapy: instrument grip, needle gripping, two-handed tying techniques, needle penetration, and suture guiding.

Microsurgical instruments are most stable when held like a writing instrument (Fig. 4.6). Needles are best gripped about two-thirds down from the end of the needle (Fig. 4.7). One technique for holding the needle is to grasp the suture with tying forceps in one's nondominant hand about 2–3 cm from the needle. Dangle the needle until it rests on the tissue and grasp the needle with the needle holder (Fig. 4.8). The needle should be set in the needle holder pointing along the intended path.

Needle penetration should be perpendicular to the incision line. The needle should penetrate and exit the tissue at equal distances (Fig. 4.9). Depending on the needle diameter, the proper amount of tissue to engage is approximately 2 times that of the diameter of the needle. Engaging large amounts of tissue may not result in proper closure. The suture is best pulled through the tissue in a straight line perpendicular to the incision. Tying forceps can aid in this maneuver (Fig. 4.10).

Three common techniques are used in microsurgical tying: nondominant, dominant, and a combination of the two. These techniques are best learned in a laboratory setting

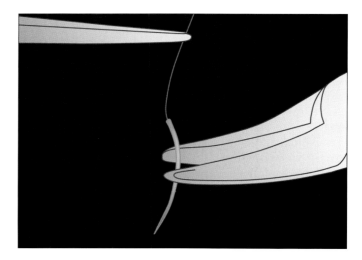

Figure 4.8. Rearming of needle.

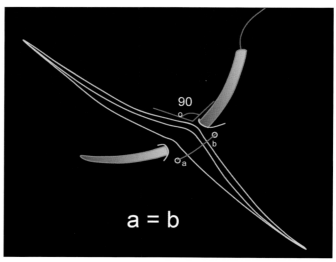

Figure 4.9. Proper entry and exit distance of needle.

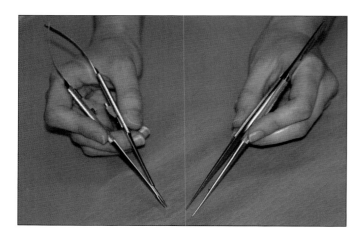

Figure 4.6. Pen grip used for microsurgical instruments.

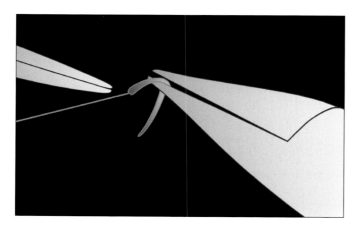

Figure 4.7. Proper gripping of needle by needle holder.

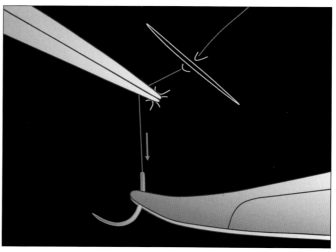

Figure 4.10. Guiding the suture direction with tying forceps.

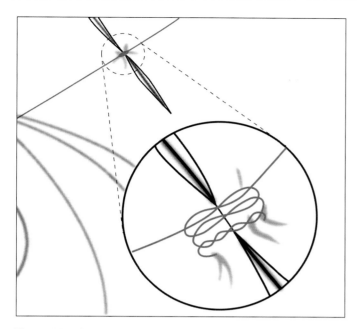

Figure 4.11. Microsurgical knot (surgeon's knot followed by square knot).

and are well referenced and described in detail in *A Laboratory Manual for Microvascular and Microtubal Surgery* (Cooley 2001). The nondominant and combination tying techniques are the two most commonly used in dentistry.

Square knots are the best to guarantee the integrity of the knot. A surgeon's knot followed by a square knot is the preferred knot combination (Fig. 4.11). Adding excess ties to a knot does not increase its strength or integrity; it only adds to the bulk of the knot.

PERIODONTAL MICROSURGICAL PROCEDURES

Mucogingival procedures

Early attempts at root coverage included lateral flaps, free gingival grafts, and coronal advanced flaps, but the results of these methods were often unpredictable. In 1985, Raetzke published a new method for covering localized areas of root exposure described as the connective tissue graft.

A comparative summary of root-coverage studies (Greenwell et al. 2000) concluded that the connective tissue graft was the most effective and predictable method. Furthermore, another comparative study of connective tissue grafts using microsurgical and macrosurgical techniques showed substantially improved vascularization of the grafts and the percentage of root coverage compared with the conventional macroscopic approach (Burdhardt & Land 2005).

Microsurgical techniques for connective tissue grafts

Several macrosurgical techniques have been outlined in the literature for connective tissue graft recipient sites. These techniques were described as a "box" or flap, and sulcular and laterally positioned flaps over the connective tissue graft. Langer & Langer (1989) were two authors who described one of the earlier approaches for connective tissue grafts. The refinements to this conventional procedure using microsurgical techniques allow for better positioning and closure of the incisions and, according to Burdhardt & Land (2005), better results.

Another approach to treat minimal recession is to use a sulcular, or flapless, technique. After the root is prepared with citric acid and/or tetracycline, a sulcular incision is made to detach the tissue by using a crescent knife, which, in turn, creates a pouch to receive the graft. The graft is sized at approximately 3 mm wider and longer than the recession defect and placed into the pouch.

The sling technique for microsurgical suturing is used to intimately familiarize the graft to the root surface. A 7-0 or 8-0 suture and a spatula needle are used for this portion of the procedure. The needle is first passed through the sulcus, then inverted and passed through the graft, and finally out through the interproximal tissue (Fig. 4.11). As the suture is tied, the graft is tightened against the root, enabling intimate stabilization. This technique is effective in recession depths of 3 mm or less.

Numerous other microsurgical techniques can be used, such as tunnel techniques, or lateral flaps covering the connective graft in more advanced recession cases (more than 3 mm). These techniques are similar to macrosurgical flap design, but are more refined because of smaller instrumentation, needles, and sutures.

Microsurgical applications for root preparation

Stereomicroscopy has often been used in dentistry to evaluate residual calculus after scaling and surgical therapy. Several researchers believe the critical determinant of successful periodontal therapy is the thoroughness of debridement of the root surface (Lindhe & Nyman 1984; Lindhe et al. 1984). Fleischer et al. (1989) stated that, regardless of the experience level of the operator, calculus-free roots were obtained more often with surgical access. Other articles comparing the amount of residual calculus on root surfaces treated by scaling and root preparation showed less residual calculus on those treated with surgical access (14%–24%) than on those treated without surgical access (17%–69%) (American Academy of Periodontology 1996).

Root preparation is enhanced when performed under illumination (Reinhardt et al. 1985). The surgical operating microscope is an excellent source of light. Although few studies have compared root preparation during surgical access with, and without, magnification, it seems logical that a surgical operating microscope would enhance a surgeon's effectiveness in root preparation.

INCORPORATING THE SURGICAL OPERATING MICROSCOPE INTO PRACTICE

Microsurgical skills are not beyond the ability of dentists. We often work in small and confined places. It can require numerous hours of training to use the microscope, similar to the neurological retraining we had to accomplish to switch from direct view to indirect mirror view. Certain principles of microsurgery should to be adhered to, and one should approach training in microsurgery with a fresh and open mind. One should not approach learning the skills of microsurgery as an endurance test. Frequent breaks and recurrent training are beneficial. Certainly, controlled training at a microsurgical training facility with experienced faculty speeds up the process.

Several hurdles must be overcome in microsurgical training. Tremor or intrinsic, unwanted muscle movement is a problem all operators of the surgical microscope deal with to some degree. The consensus of experienced microsurgeons is that tremors are enhanced by sleep deprivation, physical exertion of the upper body within 24 h, recent nicotine exposure, excessive caffeine, irritation, and anxiety. One should avoid these before performing microsurgery.

Another skill that takes time to learn is depth-of-field perception. Similar to adapting to different visual clues when first wearing loupes, you will need time to adjust to the new visual field through a surgical microscope.

Unless the anterior facial teeth or gingival tissues are the targets, mirrors are extremely useful. Usually they are held further away from the teeth, and smaller sizes and bent handles will facilitate technique. One should also become skilled at the positioning of the microscope.

Documentation of procedures is possible through video and digital photography. It is beyond the scope of this chapter to inform readers of what photographic systems to use. The manufacturers of the surgical operating microscopes can aid professionals in setting up such systems.

SUMMARY

The surgical operating microscope provides practitioners with increased illumination, magnification, and an environment in which surgical skills can be refined. Clinicians have smaller instrumentation, sutures, and needles at their disposal to facilitate enhanced clinical skills. Although only a few studies show enhanced surgical outcomes, the increase in visual acuity provided by the surgical operating microscope should enhance a periodontist's delivery of surgical skills.

REFERENCES

Anatol, T.I., Roopchand, R., Holder, Y., & Shing-Hon, G. (1997) A comparison of the use of plain catgut, skin tapes and polyglactin sutures for skin closure: A prospective clinical trial. *Journal of the Royal College of Surgeons of Edinborough* 42, 124–127.

Apotheker, H., & Jako, G.H. (1981) A microscope for use in dentistry. *Journal of Microsurgery* 3, 7–10.

Barraquer, J.I. (1980) The history of the microscope in ocular surgery. *Journal of Microsurgery* 1, 288–299.

Belcher, J.M. (2001) A perspective on periodontal microsurgery. *International Journal of Periodontology and Restorative Dentistry* 21, 191–196.

Burdhardt, R., & Land, N.P. (2005) Coverage of localized gingival recessions: Comparison of micro- and macrosurgical techniques. *Journal of Clinical Periodontology* 32, 287–293.

Campbell, D. (1989) Magnification is major aid to dentists . . . and how microdentistry's time has come! *Future of Dentistry* 4(3), 11.

Carr, G.B. (1992) Microscopes in endodontics. *Journal of California Dentistry* 20, 55–61.

Cobb, C.M. (1996) Non-surgical pocket therapy: Mechanical. *Annals of Periodontology* 1, 443–490.

Cooley, B.C. (2001) *A Laboratory Manual for Microsulcular and Microtubal Surgery*. Reading, PA: Surgical Specialties, 28–33.

Dohlman, G.F. (1969) Carl Olof Nylen and the birth of the otomicroscope and microsurgery. *Archives of Otolaryngology* 90, 813–817.

Fleischer, H.C., Mellonig, J.T., Brayer, W.K., Gray, J.L., & Barnett, J.D. (1989) Scaling and root planing efficacy in multirooted teeth. *Journal of Periodontology* 60, 402–409.

Greenwell, H., Bissada, N.F., Henderson, R.D., & Dodge, J.R. (2000) The deceptive nature of root coverage results. *Journal of Periodontology* 71, 1327–1337.

Johnson & Johnson (1994) *Wound Closure Manual*. Somerville, NJ: Ethicon.

LaBabnara, J. (1995) A review of absorbable suture materials in head and neck surgery and introduction of monocryl: A new absorbable suture. *Ear, Nose, and Throat Journal* 74, 409–416.

Langer, B., & Langer, L. (1989) Subepithelial connective tissue graft technique for root coverage. *Journal of Periodontology* 56, 715–720.

Leknius, C., & Geissberger, M. (1995) The effect of magnification on the performance of fixed prosthodontic procedures. *Journal of the California Dental Association* 23, 66–70.

Lindhe, J., & Nyman, S. (1984) Long-term maintenance of patients treated for advanced periodontal disease. *Journal of Clinical Periodontology* 11, 504–514.

Lindhe, J., Westfelt, E., Nyman, S., Socransky, S.S., & Haffajee, A.D. (1984) Long-term effect of surgical/nonsurgical treatment of periodontal disease. *Journal of Clinical Periodontology* 11, 448–458.

Raetzke, P.B. (1985) Covering localized areas of root exposure employing the "envelope" technique. *Journal of Periodontology* 56, 397–402.

Reinhardt, R.A., Johnson, G.K., & Tussing, G.J. (1985) Root planing with interdental papillae reflection and fiber optic illumination. *Journal of Periodontology* 56, 721–726.

Tibbetts, L.S., & Shanelec, D.A. 1998. Periodontal microsurgery. *Dental Clinics of North America* 42, 339–359.

Chapter 5: Free Gingival Autograft

Serge Dibart

HISTORY

Bjorn in 1963, and Sullivan & Atkins in 1968, were the first to describe the free gingival autograft. The latter two applied the principles of plastic surgery to periodontology. The autograft was initially used to increase the amount of attached gingiva and extend the vestibular fornix. Later it was used to attempt coverage of exposed root surfaces (Sullivan & Atkins 1968; Holbrook & Ochsenbein 1983; Miller 1985). Simple and highly predictable when used to increase the amount of attached gingiva, it is also quite versatile: it can also be used over an extraction socket or osseous graft (Ellegaard et al. 1974).

INDICATIONS

Free gingival autografts are used for:

- Increasing the amount of keratinized tissue (more specifically, attached gingiva)

- Increasing the vestibular depth

- Increasing the volume of gingival tissues in edentulous spaces (preprosthetic procedures)

- Covering roots in areas of gingival recession

ARMAMENTARIUM

This includes the basic surgical kit plus the following:

- Absorbable gelatin sponge (Gelfoam; Pharmacia Upjohn, Kalamazoo, MI, USA), oxidized regenerated cellulose (Surgicel; Johnson & Johnson, New Brunswick, NJ, USA) or Avitene (Bard, Murray Hill, NJ, USA)

- Purified n-butyl cyanoacrylate (PeriAcryl GluStitch; Delta, BC, Canada)

- Citric acid pH 1 (40%) or 1 capsule of tetracycline hydrochloride (HCl), 250 mg, for root coverage

FREE GINGIVAL AUTOGRAFT TO INCREASE KERATINIZED TISSUE

Technique

Preparation of the recipient site

Using the scalpel, a no. 15 blade, trace the horizontal incision line below the gingival recession (Figs. 5.1 & 5.2). You may keep or remove the gingival sulcus. Place two vertical incisions, extending beyond the mucogingival junction, at the end of that horizontal line. Place the releasing incisions at line angles of the adjacent teeth and proceed with a par-

tial thickness flap, leaving the periosteum on the alveolar bone.

At this stage, it is critical to dissect as close as possible to the periosteum, to remove epithelium, connective tissue, and muscle fibers, so there is as little movable soft tissue as possible. This decreases the likelihood of a movable graft after the healing process.

Once the bed has been prepared, the superficial flap can be removed using scissors. If you decide to keep the flap, it should be sutured below the graft once the graft has been secured.

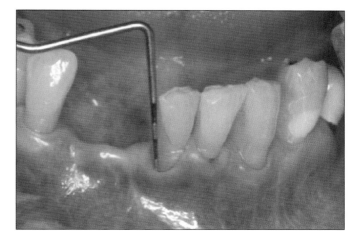

Figure 5.1. Tooth 25 had a recession and lack of attached gingiva.

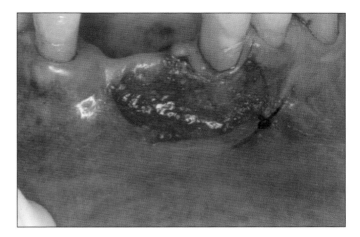

Figure 5.2. Preparation of the recipient site. A bleeding vessel has been tied with a black silk suture.

Some authors advocate the placement of the graft on denuded bone (Dordick et al. 1976; James & McFall 1978), reporting less shrinkage and a firmer, less mobile graft. In this particular technique, the surgeon removes the periosteum, as well as the other structures mentioned previously, such as the epithelium, connective tissue, and muscle fibers, to expose the alveolar bone. The incisions go down to the bone, with the blade in contact with the bone, cutting the periosteum.

The full-thickness flap is then elevated with a periosteal elevator to uncover the underlying bone. This dissection is called a *blunt dissection* as opposed to the aforementioned *sharp dissection* for the partial thickness flap. If the graft is placed on denuded bone, it is important to decorticate the alveolar plate using a small round burr (no. 1/2). This enables faster revascularization of the graft via the formation of capillary outgrowths.

Graft harvesting from the donor site

It is customary to take the graft from the palate between the palatal root of the first molar and the distal line angle of the canine. This is the area where the thickest tissue can be found (Reiser et al. 1996). However, any other edentulous area, such as the edentulous ridge, attached gingiva, or accessible tuberosities, will be just as sufficient.

When harvesting the graft, it is advisable to avoid the neurovascular bundle, which includes the greater and lesser palatine nerves and blood vessels. Avoid the palatal rugae as well (Cohen 1994). The neurovascular bundle enters the palate through the greater and lesser palatine foramina, apical to the third molars, and then travels across the palate and into the incisive foramen.

Reiser et al. in 1996 reported that the neurovascular bundle could be located 7–17 mm from the cemento-enamel junction (CEJ) of the maxillary premolars and molars. According to these authors, in the average palatal vault the distance from the CEJ to the neurovascular bundle is 12 mm (Fig. 5.3). That distance is shortened to 7 mm in case of a shallow palatal vault and lengthened to 17 mm in case of a high palatal vault.

Other research has shown gender-related variations. The mean height of the palatal vault, as measured from the midline of the palate to the CEJ of the first molars, is 14.90 ± 2.93 mm in men and 12.70 ± 2.45 mm in women (Redman et al. 1965).

Needle sounding while anesthetizing the area can be a useful tool in approximating the location of the palatal artery as well as the thickness of the tissues. The inclusion of palatal rugae in the graft should be avoided because it could be detrimental to aesthetics. The transplanted graft

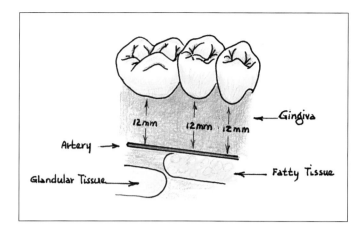

Figure 5.3. Anatomy of a donor region. Palatal vessels and nerve running from the greater and lesser palatine foramina to the interincisive foramen. The anterior palatal submucosa is mainly fatty, whereas the posterior palatal submucosa is mainly glandular.

may retain its original morphology long after the procedure is done, and the rugae remain despite efforts to eliminate them surgically (Breault et al. 1999).

After measuring the denuded area with a periodontal probe at the recipient site, the measurements of the palate should be recorded and the graft outline traced with the scalpel (Fig. 5.4). The graft thickness should be close to 1.5 mm, which approximately corresponds to the length of the bevel on a no. 15 blade, and should not be too thick or too thin. The dissection is done with a no. 15 blade kept parallel to the epithelial outer side of the graft, not the long axis of the tooth.

The submucosa of the anterior palate is rich in fat (Orban 1996) and care must be taken to avoid including the fatty layer in the graft. If that layer is included, the fat is removed from the graft with the scalpel before suturing it to the

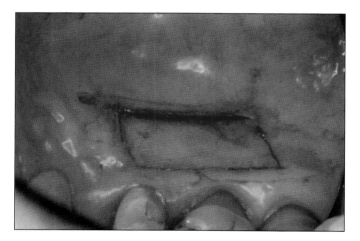

Figure 5.4. Palatal donor site. The graft to be harvested had been delineated with a no. 15 blade.

recipient bed. The excision has to be atraumatic, and every effort must be made to have a smooth, even, and regular connective tissue surface (Figs. 5.5 & 5.6). This is important because it will minimize dead space between the graft and the recipient bed and enable quick revascularization of the graft.

Once the graft is harvested, it should be immediately sutured onto the recipient site with the connective tissue facing down against the periosteum of the recipient site.

Graft suturing

The use of resorbable or nonresorbable material is a matter of personal preference. Silk is easy to use but should be removed after 1 week. Gut/chromic gut, on the other hand, will resorb in 1–2 weeks. Single interrupted sutures are usually placed to secure the graft mesially and distally (Fig. 5.7). A mesiodistal horizontal suture could be added to wrap the lower half of the graft (Fig. 5.8). Variations include intraperiosteal X sutures (Fig. 5.9). They are all

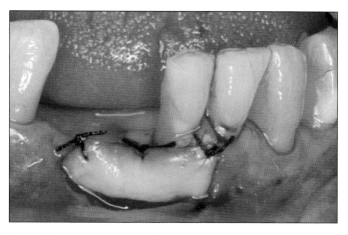

Figure 5.7. The graft is sutured in place with three single interrupted silk sutures (5-0). At this stage, when pulling on the lip, the graft should be immobile.

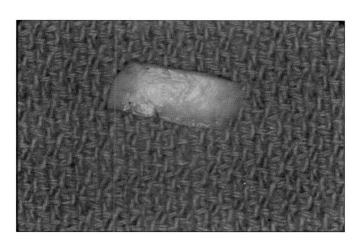

Figure 5.5. The palatal graft has been harvested.

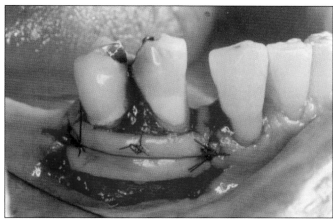

Figure 5.8. The mesiodistal horizontal suture.

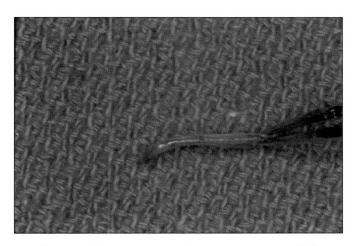

Figure 5.6. The graft is even and approximately 1.5 mm thick.

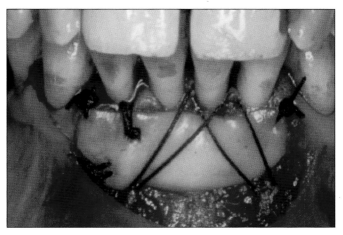

Figure 5.9. The graft is kept in place by adding two circular intraperiosteal sutures to the four single interrupted sutures present.

aimed at immobilizing the graft and decreasing the amount of dead space between recipient site and graft. This helps minimize the size of the blood clot and creates a better adaptation that will ensure prompt and proper revascularization.

Applying some pressure with wet gauze over the sutured graft for a few minutes will displace the blood under the graft, reducing hematomas, and closely position the graft to the recipient bed. Plasma will be converted to fibrin, and this fibrin clot will anchor the graft to its bed and enable rapid penetration by capillaries. It will act as a matrix through which metabolites and waste products diffuse (Foman 1960). A good test for checking the immobility of the graft is to pull the lip or cheek gently once the graft has been sutured. If the graft moves, then the suturing or the size of the recipient bed was inadequate.

A small periodontal dressing is applied on the graft to protect the recipient site. Care must be taken when applying the dressing so it will not impinge on occlusal surfaces; otherwise, it will be lost within hours.

Donor site

This is usually left without a dressing, so that it may granulate (Figs. 5.10 & 5.11). If the graft is large and the thickness important, it can be useful, for the comfort of the patient, to apply a piece of Gelfoam or Surgicel to the donor site and suture over it with X sutures. This is followed by an application of a few drops of medical-grade cyanoacrylate glue (PeriAcryl), which will ensure hemostasis and decrease postoperative discomfort for the patient.

Graft healing

Prior to reestablishment of vascularization (24–48 h), the graft is solely dependent on diffusion from its host bed. This

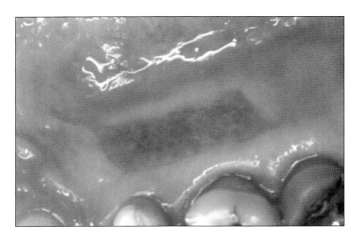

Figure 5.11. The donor site 1 week later.

diffusion, which is called *plasmic circulation*, occurs most efficiently through the fibrin clot (Foman 1960; Reese & Stark 1961). The next step is the reestablishment of graft vascularization. Capillary proliferations begin at the end of day 1, and by day 2 or 3 some capillaries have extended into the graft and others have anastomosed or penetrated the graft's vasculature. Adequate blood supply does not appear to be present until about day 8 (Davis & Traut 1925).

Concomitant with vascularization, organic connective tissue union between the graft and its bed starts on day 4 and is complete by day 10. This will be responsible for the secondary contraction of the graft. Upon healing, the graft may shrink by as much as 33% (Egli et al. 1975) (Fig. 5.12).

Possible complications

The main complication of the procedure is bleeding from the donor site. This can happen during the procedure or after the patient's departure from the office.

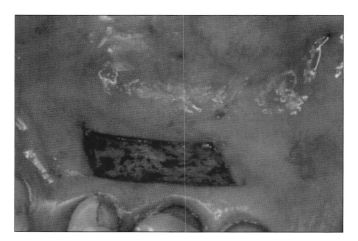

Figure 5.10. The donor site at time of surgery. The connective tissue is left exposed to granulate.

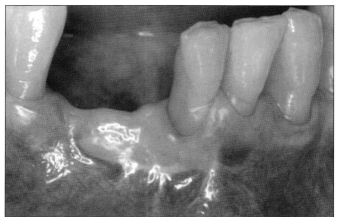

Figure 5.12. Results 2 years later. A band of attached gingival is present below and around tooth 25.

During the procedure

Do not panic if bleeding occurs during the procedure. Assess the bleeding source (arterial versus venous) and location. If the palatal artery or a branch has been severed, it is best to place one or more compressive sutures in the palate, proximal to the bleeding site, to reduce or stop the hemorrhage (Fig. 5.13). The sutures should be placed between the bleeding site and the palatal foramina.

It is useful at this stage to use a few drops of Xylocaine (lidocaine) 2% with 1/50,000 epinephrine in infiltration around the bleeding area to help with the hemostasis. Finish the grafting procedure, cover the donor site with Gelfoam or Surgicel, and secure with an X suture. Use compression with wet gauze for 5–10 min and finish by applying a few drops of PeriAcryl over the donor site.

Another alternative is to cauterize the bleeding vessel. As a last resort, some authors have advocated the elevation of a full-thickness flap to enable the visualization and ligation of the blood vessels (Hollingshead 1968).

After the procedure

If bleeding occurs after the procedure, assure the patient of his or her safety. Have the patient moisten a tea bag and ask him or her to put the tea bag on the palate and press on it for 10–15 min. If the bleeding does not stop, ask the patient to come to your office. Once in the office, use the aforementioned procedure—infiltration with lidocaine 2% with 1/50,000 epinephrine, compressive sutures, Gelfoam, etc.—or send the patient to an emergency room.

Other complications

Swelling and bruising

Another complication of the procedure may include swelling and bruising at the recipient site. After the initial use of cold pad within the first 24 h, the application of warm pads, in conjunction with anti-inflammatory medications, will ease the problem.

Graft mobility

Graft mobility after complete healing is usually the result of improper bed preparation. Too much loose tissue or muscle fibers left above the periosteum will result in graft mobility. At this point, it is not necessary to redo the graft. Raising a partial thickness flap that includes the graft, removing the loose tissues above the periosteum, and resuturing generally solve the problem.

VARIATION ON THE SAME THEME: FREE CONNECTIVE TISSUE GRAFT

Use of a de-epithelialized graft can increase the amount of attached gingiva (Edel 1974). The gingiva is reported to be stable at 6 months with a mean contraction of 28%. There is complete epithelialization of the connective tissue surface at 2 weeks, with the graft blending into the surrounding tissues at 6 weeks.

FREE GINGIVAL AUTOGRAFT FOR ROOT COVERAGE

Technique

The technique and armamentarium of the free gingival autograft for root coverage are basically the same as the free gingival autograft to increase keratinized tissue with the addition of the steps listed next (Figs. 5.14–5.17).

Preparation of the recipient site

After anesthesia, thorough root planning of the recession by using a Gracey curette or back-action chisel is recommended. This removes the contaminated cementum and flattens the root surface, if necessary. Any concavity or

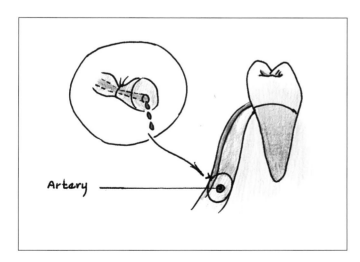

Figure 5.13. Compressive suture of the palatal artery.

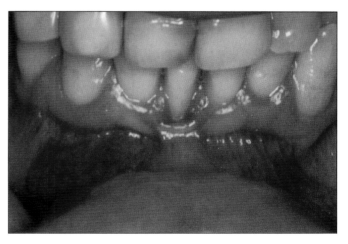

Figure 5.14. Free gingival graft for root coverage.

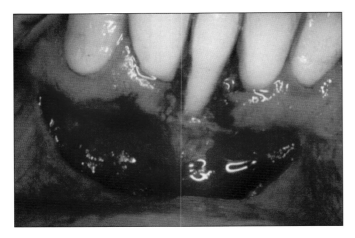

Figure 5.15. A large periosteal bed is prepared to receive the graft. The large size of the bed is to compensate for the avascular area of the root to be covered and eliminate frenum fiber attachment.

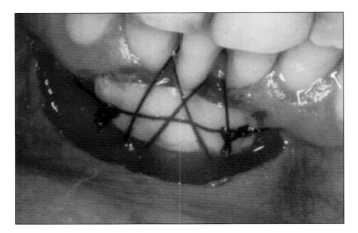

Figure 5.16. The palatal graft is sutured to the recipient bed by using a mesiodistal horizontal suture and two circular intraperiosteal sutures.

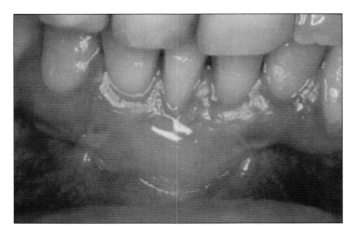

Figure 5.17. The area 1 year later. Take note of the root coverage on tooth 25, the amount of keratinized gingiva, and the absence of labial frenum pull.

convexity on the root surface should be eliminated or reduced at this stage by using hand or rotary instruments.

Immediately after root planning, saturated citric acid is burnished into the root surface for 5 min by using cotton pellets (Miller 1985). An alternative to citric acid is tetracycline HCl, 50–100 mg/ml, for 3–5 min. This opens the dentinal tubules (Polson et al. 1984) and removes the smear layer that could act as a barrier to the connective tissue attachment to the root surface (Isik et al. 2000). The area is rinsed thoroughly, and horizontal incisions are made at the level of the CEJ, preserving the interdental papillae.

This is followed by vertical incisions at least one tooth away from each side of the recession. This point is critical, because the portion of the free gingival graft placed over the denuded root will not survive if there is not a recipient bed large enough to provide collateral vascularization. Therefore, the bed should be as wide as possible, given the anatomical limitation of the area. It should extend apically at least 3 mm below the margin of the denuded root. The wider the bed, the better chance the patient has for root coverage.

Graft healing

This includes all of the aforementioned steps plus the advent of a creeping attachment, as described by Matter (1980). This phenomenon provides additional root coverage during healing, which may be observed between 1 month and 1 year after grafting. An average of 1.2 mm of coronal creep at 1 year has been reported (Matter 1980).

REFERENCES

Bjorn, H. (1963) Free transplantation of gingival propria. *Svensk Tandlakare Tidskrift* 22, 684–685.

Breault, L.G., Fowler, E.B., & Billman, M.A. (1999) Retained free gingival graft rugae: A 9-year case report. *Journal of Periodontology* 70, 438–440.

Cohen, E.S. (1994) *Atlas of Cosmetic and Reconstructive Periodontal Surgery.* Philadelphia: Lea and Febiger.

Davis, J.S., & Traut, H.F. (1925) Origin and development of the blood supply of whole-thickness skin grafts. *Annals of Surgery* 82, 871–879.

Dordick, B., Coslet, J.G., & Seibert, J.S. (1976) Clinical evaluation of free autogenous gingival grafts placed on alveolar bone. *Journal of Periodontology* 41, 559–567.

Edel, A. (1974) Clinical evaluation of free connective tissue grafts used to increase the width of keratinized tissue. *Journal of Clinical Periodontology* 1, 185–196.

Egli, U., Vollmer, W., & Rateitschak, K.H. (1975) Follow-up studies of free gingival grafts. *Journal of Clinical Periodontology* 2, 98–104.

Ellegaard, B., Karring, T., & Loe, H. (1974) New periodontal attachment procedure based on retardation of epithelial migration. *Journal of Clinical Periodontology* 1, 75–88.

Foman, S. (1960) *Cosmetic Surgery.* Philadelphia: Lippincott.

Holbrook, T., & Ochsenbein, C. (1983) Complete coverage of the denuded root surface with a one stage gingival graft. *International Journal of Periodontics and Restorative Dentistry* 3(3), 9–27.

Hollingshead, W.H. (1968) *The Head and Neck Anatomy for Surgeons,* vol. 1, 2nd edition. Hagerstown, MD: Harper & Row.

Isik, A.G., Tarim, B., Hafez, A.A., Yalcin, F.S., Onan, U., & Cox, C.F. (2000) A comparative scanning electron microscopic study on the characteristics of demineralized dentin root surface using different tetracycline HCl concentrations and application times. *Journal of Periodontology* 71, 219–225.

James, W.C., & McFall, W.T. (1978) Placement of free gingival grafts on denuded alveolar bone. *Journal of Periodontology* 49, 283–290.

Matter, J. (1980) Creeping attachment of free gingival grafts: A 5-year follow-up study. *Journal of Periodontology* 51, 681–685.

Miller, P.D. (1985) Root coverage using the free soft tissue autograft following citric acid application. III. A successful and predictable procedure in areas of deep wide recession. *International Journal of Periodontics and Restorative Dentistry* 5(2), 15–37.

Orban, B.J. (1996) *Oral Histology and Embryology,* 6th edition. Edited by H. Sicher. St. Louis: C.V. Mosby.

Polson, A.M., Frederick, G.T., Ladenheim, S., & Hanes, P.J. (1984) The production of a root surface smear layer by instrumentation and its removal by citric acid. *Journal of Periodontology* 55, 443–446.

Redman, R.S., Shapiro, B.L., & Gonlin, R.J. (1965) Measurement of normal and reportedly malformed palatal vaults. II. Normal juvenile measurements. *Journal of Dental Research* 45, 266–267.

Reese, J.D., & Stark, R.B. (1961) Principles of free skin grafting. *Bulletin of New York Academy of Medicine* (Ser 2) 37, 213.

Reiser, G.M., Bruno, J.F., Mahan, P.E., & Larkin, L.H. (1996) The subepithelial connective tissue graft palatal donor site: Anatomic considerations for surgeons. *International Journal of Periodontics and Restorative Dentistry* 16, 131–137.

Sullivan, H., & Atkins, J. (1968) Free autogenous gingival grafts. I. Principles of successful grafting. *Periodontics* 6, 121–129.

Chapter 6: Subepithelial Connective Tissue Graft

Serge Dibart and Mamdouh Karima

HISTORY

First described in the literature in 1985 (Langer & Langer 1985; Raetzke 1985) as a predictable means for root coverage, a subepithelial connective tissue graft combines the use of a partial thickness flap with the placement of a connective tissue graft. This enables the graft to benefit from a double vascularization, from both the periosteum and the buccal flap.

In addition, the connective tissue carries the genetic message for the overlying epithelium to be keratinized (Edel 1974). Therefore, only connective tissue from a keratinized mucosa should be used as a graft. The partial thickness flap may or may not have vertical releasing incisions (Langer & Langer 1985; Raetzke 1985; Bruno 1994).

Vertical releasing incisions will noticeably reduce the blood supply of the flap. The gingiva is vascularized from the apical area, the interdental septum, and the periosteum. An envelope or a pouch design, without the vertical incisions, has a better likelihood for success than does a flap with vertical releasing incisions. The advantages of the technique are the maintenance of the blood supply to the flap, a close adaptation to the graft, and reduction in postoperative discomfort and scarring.

The predictability and superior aesthetics provided by this technique make it the gold standard for root coverage. Jahnke et al. (1993) reported a success rate fivefold greater for achieving 100% root coverage when using a connective tissue graft versus a thick free gingival graft.

INDICATIONS

- Root coverage in areas of gingival recession (mild, moderate, or severe)
- Gingival coverage of exposed implant abutment or metal collar.
- Increase in the width of attached gingiva
- Ridge augmentation (edentulous area)

ARMAMENTARIUM

This includes the basic surgical kit plus citric acid pH 1 (40%) or one capsule of tetracycline hydrochloride (HCl) 250 mg.

TECHNIQUE (ENVELOPE FLAP)

Preparation of the recipient site

Root coverage

After anesthesia, thorough root planning of the recession by using a Gracey curette (Hu-Friedy, Chicago, IL, USA) or back-action chisel is recommended. This will remove the contaminated cementum and flatten the root surface, if necessary. Any concavity or convexity on the root surface should be eliminated or reduced at this stage by using hand or rotary instruments.

Immediately after root planning, saturated citric acid is burnished into the root surface for 5 min by using cotton pellets (Miller 1985). An alternative to citric acid is tetracycline HCl (50–100 mg/ml for 3–5 min). This will open the dentinal tubules (Polson 1984) and remove the smear layer that could act as a barrier to the connective tissue attachment from the root surface (Isik 2000).

Gingival coverage of an implant collar

Clean the metal collar thoroughly by using a cotton pellet soaked with tetracycline HCl (100 mg/ml). There is no need to scale the exposed collar (Fig. 6.1)

Incisions and creation of the "pouch"

The technique is similar for root coverage or implant coverage.

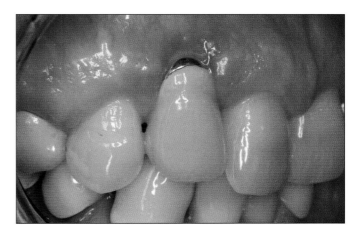

Figure 6.1. The metal collar of the implant showing compromised aesthetics.

The area is rinsed thoroughly and a horizontal incision is made from cemento-enamel junction (CEJ) to CEJ on each side of the gingival recession with a no. 15 blade. The blade is then kept almost parallel to the long axis of the tooth, with the blade tip aimed at the underlying bone to keep the buccal flap from perforating.

A pouch is created through sharp dissection, which has to be carried beyond the mucogingival line to mobilize the buccal flap to reach the CEJ coronally. The pouch is ready when a periodontal probe placed below the recession can coronally move the buccal flap to the CEJ without trouble.

Harvesting the graft from the donor site

Two parallel incisions, perpendicular to the long axis of the teeth, are made in the palate, close to the CEJ (Langer & Langer 1985). Two vertical releasing incisions help dissect the superficial flap and free the subepithelial connective tissue graft (Fig. 6.2). Stay within the safety zone, anterior to the palatal root of the first molar and within 12 mm of the CEJ. Once the graft is harvested, the success rate of the procedure does not appear to be influenced by removing the epithelial collar from the graft (Bouchard et al. 1994).

Suturing of the graft

The graft is inserted in the subepithelial space created beneath the flap (Fig. 6.3). The coronal portion of the graft lies at, or slightly above, the CEJ level, and the graft is secured to the papillae by using resorbable single inter-rupted sutures. The buccal flap is then pulled upward over the graft with a sling suture (Fig. 6.4). This helps give the graft maximal buccal coverage and ensure optimal vascularization.

It is useful at this stage to insert the curved end of a periosteal elevator (24G or Pritchard) (Hu-Friedy) between the graft and the flap prior to suturing. This will guide the

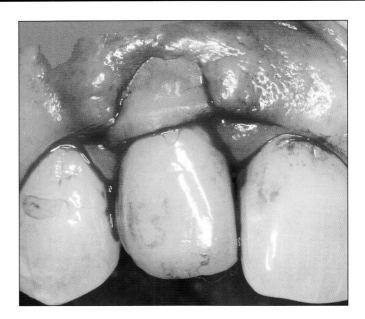

Figure 6.3. The envelope flap (pouch) has been created and the connective tissue graft inserted.

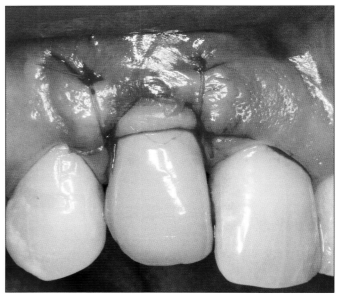

Figure 6.4. The graft is sutured to the papillae, and the buccal flap is sutured over the graft by using a sling suture. It is important to cover as much of the graft as possible to maximize vascular supply.

needle when suturing the buccal flap. The needle slides on the elevator and does not engage the graft, enabling the buccal flap to move upward and cover the graft as much as possible. Wet gauze is applied with mild pressure on the wound to minimize dead space between the recipient site, the graft, and the flap. A periodontal dressing is applied on the graft and left for 1 week. The healing is usually uneventful and the results predictable (Figs. 6.5–6.7).

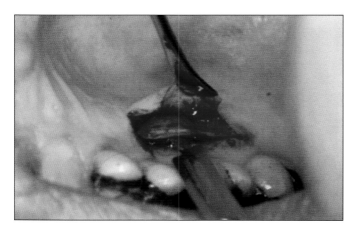

Figure 6.2. The trapdoor enabling the retrieval of the connective tissue graft.

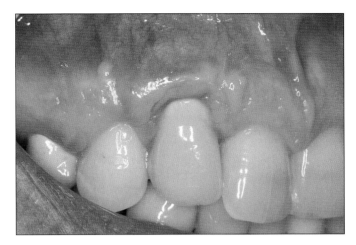

Figure 6.5. After 3 months, the aesthetics have been improved tremendously by the procedure.

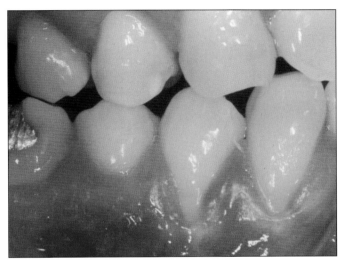

Figure 6.6. A Miller class II gingival recession affecting teeth 27 and 28.

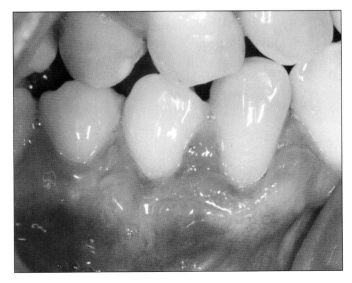

Figure 6.7. Results of 100% root coverage 3 weeks after periodontal microsurgery.

Suturing of the donor site

Suture the palatal flap back into position immediately after taking the donor tissue; this will reduce the size of the blood clot, which could cause tissue necrosis. Homeostasis is best accomplished with horizontal mattress sutures in the following way: the sutures (a) pass through a mesial interproximal space on the buccal surface, (b) penetrate the palatal mucosa apical and distal to the base of the graft site, (c) exit the palate mesially, and (d) cross to the distal interproximal space to be tied on the buccal surface.

This method of suturing compresses the palatal flap, approximates the wound edges (primary intention healing), and provides homeostasis. Since there is no denuded palatal area, the patient reports less postoperative discomfort than with a free gingival graft and less risk of postoperative bleeding. Dressing on the palate is optional.

Possible complication

It is bleeding (please refer to Chapter 5).

REFERENCES

Bouchard, P., Etienne, D., Ouhayoun, J.P., & Nilveus, R. (1994) Subepithelial connective tissue grafts in the treatment of gingival recessions: A comparative study of two procedures. *Journal of Periodontology* 65, 929–936.

Bruno, J.F. (1994) Connective tissue graft technique assuring wide root coverage. *International Journal of Periodontics and Restorative Dentistry* 14, 127–137.

Edel, A. (1974) Clinical evaluation of free connective tissue grafts used to increase the width of keratinized gingiva. *Journal of Clinical Periodontology* 1, 185–196.

Isik, A.G., Tarim, B., Hafez, A.A., Yalcin, F.S., Onan, U., & Cox, C.F. (2000) A comparative scanning electron microscopic study on the characteristics of demineralized dentin root surface using different tetracycline HCl concentrations and application times. *Journal of Periodontology* 71, 219–225.

Jahnke, P.V., Sandifer, J.B., Gher, M.E., Gray, J.L., & Richardson, A.C. (1993) Thick free gingival and connective tissue autografts for root coverage. *Journal of Periodontology* 64, 315–322.

Langer, B., & Langer, L. (1985) Subepithelial connective tissue graft technique for root coverage. *Journal of Periodontology* 56, 715–720.

Miller, P.D. (1985) Root coverage using the free soft tissue autograft following citric acid application. III. A successful and predictable procedure in areas of deep wide recession. *International Journal of Periodontics and Restorative Dentistry* 5(2), 15–37.

Polson, A.M., Frederick, G.T., Ladenheim, S., & Hanes, P.J. (1984) The production of a root surface smear layer by instrumentation and its removal by citric acid. *Journal of Periodontology* 55, 443–446.

Raetzke, P.B. (1985) Covering localized areas of root exposure employing the "envelope" technique. *Journal of Periodontology* 56, 397–402

Chapter 7: Pedicle Grafts: Rotational Flaps and Double-Papilla Procedure

Serge Dibart and Mamdouh Karima

HISTORY

Grupe & Warren were the first to describe the sliding flap as a method to repair isolated gingival defects (1956). They reported elevating a full-thickness flap one tooth away from the defect and rotating it to cover the recession. In 1967, Hattler reported the use of a sliding partial thickness flap to correct mucogingival defects on two or three adjacent teeth.

In 1968, Cohen & Ross, using the interproximal papillae to cover recessions and correct gingival defects in areas of insufficient gingiva not suitable for a lateral sliding flap, described the double-papilla repositioned flap. This technique offers the advantages of dual blood supply and denudation of interdental bone only, which is less susceptible to permanent damage after surgical exposure. A full-thickness or partial thickness flap may be used. The latter is preferable because it offers the advantage of quicker healing in the donor site and reduces the risk of facial bone height loss, particularly if the bone is thin or the presence of a dehiscence or a fenestration is suspected (Wood et al. 1972).

Indeed, Wood et al. (1972) reported increased bone at healing time with a partial thickness flap as opposed to a full-thickness flap (0.98 mm versus 0.62 mm). The advantage of the pedicle graft versus the free gingival autograft is the presence of its own blood supply, in the base, that will nourish the graft and facilitate the reestablishment of vascular anastomoses at the recipient site during the healing phase.

INDICATIONS

- Inadequate amount of attached gingiva
- Single or multiple adjacent recessions that have adequate donor tissue laterally (root coverage)
- Recession next to an edentulous area

PREREQUISITES

- Thick periodontal biotype
- Preferably deep vestibule

ARMAMENTARIUM

This includes the basic surgical kit for the lateral sliding and obliquely rotated flaps. For the double papilla, add:

- Tetracycline hydrochloride 250-mg capsule

- Gracey (Hu-Friedy, Chicago, IL, USA) curette no. 1/2
- Scalpel handle mounted with surgical blade no. 15C
- Wide-field surgical loupes (×4.5)
- Titanium instruments for microsurgery:
  - Two straight forceps
  - One straight strong forceps
  - One curved needle holder with lock
  - One straight scissors
- P-1 needle with a 7-0 coated vicryl suture

LATERAL SLIDING FLAP

Technique

After proper anesthesia (Fig. 7.1), the tissue bordering the defect is trimmed free of sulcular epithelium with a blade no. 15 and the root(s) thoroughly planned. When there is enough gingival thickness, a partial thickness flap twice as wide as the defect is reflected beyond the mucogingival junction (Fig. 7.2). The flap is then moved laterally to cover the exposed root, leaving the donor site exposed. The latter is covered by the periosteum/connective tissue (partial thickness flap) or bare bone (full-thickness flap). The flap is then secured using 5-0 single interrupted sutures (Fig. 7.3).

It is sometimes necessary to make a short oblique releasing incision at the base of the flap to avoid any tension that may impair the vascular circulation when the flap is positioned.

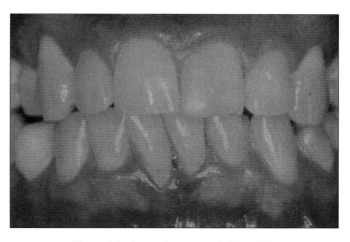

Figure 7.1. Recessions on teeth 24 and 25.

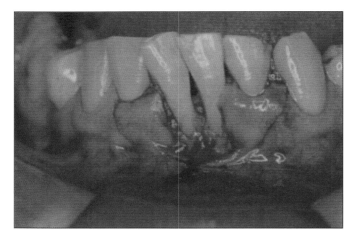

Figure 7.2. Two lateral pedicle flaps are raised adjacent to the receding areas.

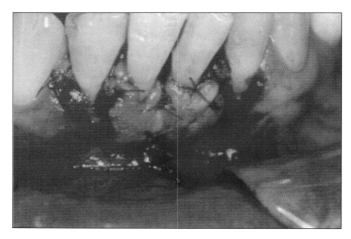

Figure 7.3. The two partial thickness lateral pedicle flaps are sutured covering the exposed root surfaces of teeth 24 and 25.

This enables the flap to lie flat and firm without excess tension at the base. Pressure is exercised on the flap with fingers and wet gauze to minimize blood clot thickness and encourage fibrinous adhesion. A periodontal dressing is applied on the wound and left in place for 1 week.

A word of caution

When operating on the lower mandible in the premolar region, take care not to injure the mental nerve. To avoid this injury, take a preoperative periapical radiograph of the area that will help locate the mental foramen, which is usually located between the first and second premolars, halfway between the alveolar crest and the lower border of the mandible. Traumatizing or severing the mental nerve can cause temporary or permanent lip and gingival paresthesia. Using a full-thickness flap approach will help minimize this possibility because a blunt dissection is used,

and the emergence of the neurovascular bundle from the mental foramen during dissection can be seen.

Wound healing

The laterally positioned flap will be healing with an attachment to the exposed root (Fig. 7.4). This attachment may be a connective tissue attachment, a long junctional epithelium, or a combination of the two (Wilderman & Wentz 1965). Avoid probing or scaling that area for 6 months. Coverage of the exposed root surfaces with this technique has varied from 60% to 72% (Albano et al. 1969; Smukler 1976; Guinnard & Caffesse 1978).

Possible complications

The most common complication is a slight recession at the donor site. This is most likely to occur if the periodontium is thin (thin biotype), with thin gingiva and thin underlying alveolar bone.

Another complication is necrosis or loosening of the flap. This happens if the flap is too thin, in a partial thickness flap, because of faulty technique or inadequate anatomy. The flap will loosen if the dissection was insufficient, and the flap was sutured with tension.

OBLIQUELY ROTATED FLAP

This is a variation of the laterally positioned flap (Pennel et al. 1965). The pedicle is rotated obliquely (90°) and sutured to the underlying connective tissue bed.

DOUBLE-PAPILLA PROCEDURE

Technique

Root surface conditioning

Use a Gracey curette no. 1/2 for scaling and root planning to treat the diseased root surface to make it biologically compatible with a healthy periodontium (Jones & O'Leary

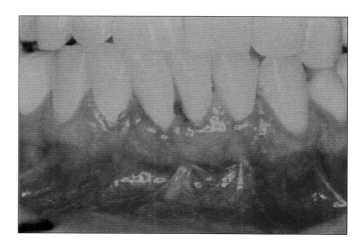

Figure 7.4. The area 1 year later.

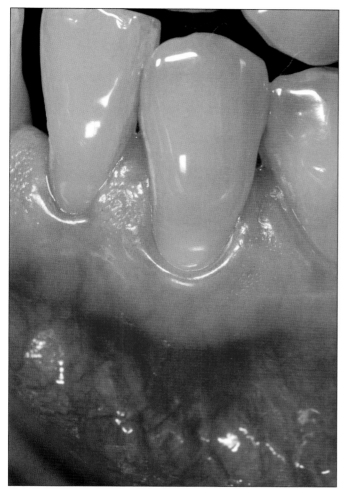

Figure 7.5. Moderate gingival recession affecting the canine.

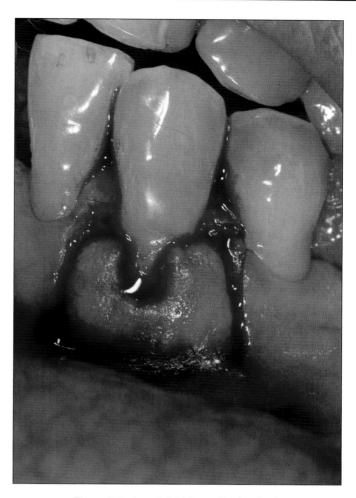

Figure 7.6. A partial thickness flap is raised.

1978) (Fig. 7.5). This includes removing the endotoxins, bacteria, and other antigens found in the cementum of the root surface.

Another form of root conditioning is performed by topical application of 50 mg/ml tetracycline for 5 min (Wikesjö et al. 1986). This is accomplished by dissolving the content of a 250-mg tetracycline capsule in 5 ml saline. Using a Q-tip, apply the tetracycline mix on the root surface and then thoroughly irrigate the root surface with water and dry it with air.

Preparation of the recipient and donor sites

Two horizontal incisions are made on both sides, parallel to the cemento-enamel junction of the tooth to be treated with a no. 15C blade. Vertical incisions are made on the mesial and the distal aspects at the surgical site and placed at the line angles of adjacent teeth (Fig. 7.6). The releasing incision is extended into alveolar mucosa without making contact with the bone.

A scalloped partial thickness internal bevel incision is made in the interdental papilla with a no. 15C blade. A partial thickness pedicle flap with sufficient mesial and distal interdental papilla is prepared. The no. 15C blade is guided to the gingival margin. After the vertical incision is made, the blade should be advanced coronally from the apical of the alveolar mucosa. A partial thickness flap is prepared.

When making the incision, always hold the blade tip parallel to the gingival surface. Undermine the interdental papilla while lifting the papilla gently with the side of the blade. Separate it from the underlying connective tissue. It is important to preserve the mesiodistal width of the interdental papilla on both sides. Use the papilla flap on either end as the donor tissue. Mesially and distally displace the two papilla flaps by half a tooth. The flaps should be wider than the recipient site to cover the root and provide a broad margin for attachment to the connective tissue border around the root.

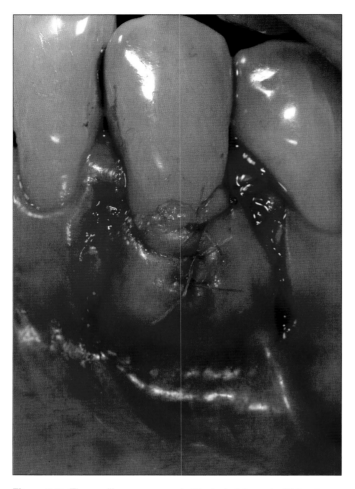

Figure 7.7. The papillae are secured with single interrupted 7.0 sutures.

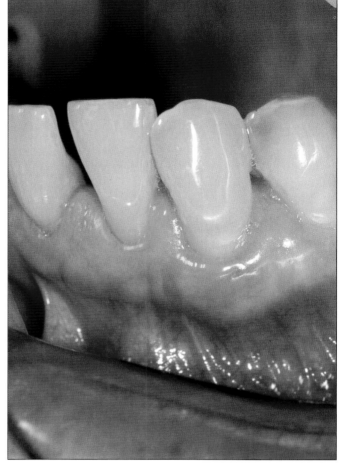

Figure 7.8. The area 2 months later.

Suturing technique

Have the ×4.5 wide-field surgical loupes on before beginning the suturing procedure. Using the microsurgical titanium straight forceps and curved needle holder with lock, suture both papilla flaps at the center of the root surface to ensure coverage of the denuded root surface. Place interrupted sutures (7-0 coated vicryl is preferred) across the medial surface of the two papilla flaps, beginning apically and working coronally. No more than two or three sutures are usually necessary. A sling suture is carried around the tooth and tied facially to prevent the graft from slipping apically (Fig. 7.7).

Apply gentle but firm pressure to the flap for 2–3 min with cotton-free gauze moistened with sterile saline solution to further secure a successful connection. To protect the surgical area during the initial phase of healing, apply a periodontal dressing, which protects the flap from displacement. The dressing must not displace the flap or impinge on its base. An improperly placed dressing may impede the blood supply to the coronal part of the flap and cause necrosis and failure.

At 1 week, the patient is instructed to use a Q-tip dipped in chlorhexidine gluconate in lieu of a toothbrush to cleanse the area. Gentle brushing of the area is initiated 2 months later (Fig. 7.8).

Possible complications

Few clinical situations would require this procedure, because many recession areas are too wide for the papilla. The only complication one might encounter, other than necrosis of the flap, is swelling and bruising at the recipient site. This is easily managed with warm pads and anti-inflammatory medications.

Suturing the two flaps over the root surface impairs blood supply, and poor results often occur using this technique. In practice, many clinicians have had limited success with the double-papilla flap. The combination connective tissue graft–double-papilla flap may increase the success rate of the procedure (Nelson 1987).

REFERENCES

Albano, E.A, Caffessee, R.C., & Carranza, F.A., Jr. (1969) A biometric analysis of laterally displaced pedicle flaps. *Revista de la Asociacion Odontologica Argentina* 57, 351–354.

Cohen, D.W., & Ross, S.E. (1968) The double papilla repositioned flap in periodontal therapy. *Journal of Periodontology* 39, 65–70.

Grupe, H.E., & Warren, R.F. (1956) Repair of gingival defects by a sliding flap operation. *Journal of Periodontology* 27, 92–95.

Guinard, E.A., & Caffesse, R.G. (1978) Treatment of localized gingival recessions. Part I. Lateral sliding flap. *Journal of Periodontology* 49, 351–356.

Hattler, A.B. (1967) Mucogingival surgery: Utilization of interdental gingiva as attached gingiva by surgical displacement. *Periodontics* 5, 126–131.

Jones, W., & O'Leary, T. (1978) The effectiveness of in vivo root planning in removing bacterial endotoxin from the roots of periodontally involved teeth. *Journal of Periodontology* 49, 337–342.

Nelson, S.W. (1987) The subepithelial connective graft: A bilaminar reconstructive procedure for the coverage of denuded root surfaces. *Journal of Periodontology* 58, 95–102.

Pennel, B.M., Higgason, J.D., Towner, J.D., King, K.O., Fritz, B.D., & Salden, J.F. (1965) Oblique rotated flap. *Journal of Periodontology* 36, 305–309.

Smukler, H. (1976) Laterally positioned mucoperiosteal pedicle grafts in the treatment of denuded roots. *Journal of Periodontology* 47, 590–595.

Wikesjö, U.M.E., Baker, P., Christersson, L., Genco, R.J., Lyall, R.M., Hic, S., DiFlorio, R.M., & Terranova, V.P. (1986) A biomedical approach to periodontal regeneration: Tetracycline treatment conditions dentin surfaces. *Journal of Periodontal Research* 21, 322–329.

Wilderman, M.N., & Wentz, F.M. (1965) Repair of a dentogingival defect with a pedicle flap. *Journal of Periodontology* 35, 218–231.

Wood, D.L., Hoag, F.M., Donnenfeld, O.W., & Rosenfeld, I.D. (1972) Alveolar crest resorption following full and partial thickness flaps. *Journal of Periodontology* 43, 141–144.

Chapter 8: Pedicle Grafts: Coronally Advanced Flaps

Serge Dibart

HISTORY

Bernimoulin et al. (1975) first reported the coronally positioned graft succeeding grafting with a free gingival autograft. This was a two-stage procedure. In the first stage, a free gingival graft was placed apical to the margins of the recession to be treated. The second stage occurred a few months later, when the graft was coronally positioned over the denuded root surfaces.

In 1986, Tarnow described the semilunar coronally positioned flap. This was a one-stage, no-suture, coronally repositioned flap aimed at correcting mild gingival recessions. In 1989, Allen and Miller reported the use of a one-stage, coronally positioned flap associated with citric acid root conditioning aimed at correcting shallow marginal recessions (2.5–4.0 mm).

INDICATIONS

A pedicle graft is used to cover gingival recessions affecting natural teeth. In the case of mild recessions, the one-stage, coronally positioned flap technique is sufficient. When the recession is moderate to severe (≥4 mm), a two-stage procedure will bring more predictable, long-term results.

Maynard (1977) outlined the following requirements as criteria for success when using coronally positioned flaps:

- The presence of shallow crevicular depths on proximal surfaces
- Normal interproximal bone heights
- Tissue height within 1 mm of the cemento-enamel junction of adjacent teeth
- Six-week healing of the free gingival graft prior to coronal positioning
- Reduction in root prominence
- Adequate release of the flap during the second-stage surgery to prevent retraction during healing

ARMAMENTARIUM

This includes the basic surgical kit plus the following:

- Gelfoam (Pharmacia-Upjohn, Kalamazoo, MI, USA) or Surgicel (Johnson & Johnson, New Brunswick, NJ, USA) (for the two-stage procedure)
- PeriAcryl (GluStitch; Delta, BC, Canada) (for the two-stage procedure)
- Citric acid, pH 1 (40%), or 1 capsule of tetracycline hydrochloride (HCl), 250 mg

CORONALLY POSITIONED FLAP: TWO STAGES

Technique

First stage

The first part of a two-stage, coronally positioned flap is a free gingival autograft (see Chapter 5) (Figs. 8.1 & 8.2).

Second stage

After a minimum 3 months of healing, the gingival graft is coronally positioned to cover the root, which should be carefully planned and conditioned with citric acid or tetracycline HCl (50–100 mg/ml) for 3–5 min. If the root has a

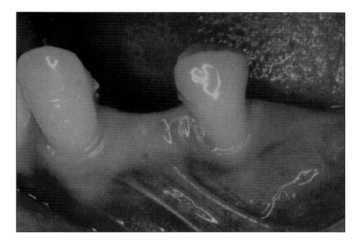

Figure 8.1. Tooth 20 has gingival recession and no attached gingiva.

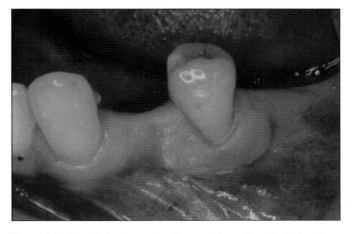

Figure 8.2. Tooth 20 at 2 months after receiving a free-gingival graft, first-step procedure.

proeminent concavity or convexity, it should be eliminated or reduced with a back-action chisel or a burr to graft on a flat surface.

The second stage requires a split-thickness dissection with mesial and distal vertical releasing incisions (Fig. 8.3). The vertical incisions are made at the line angles of the adjacent teeth when there is a full dentition and are coronally connected (horizontal intrasulcular incision). The partial thickness pedicle flap, staying close to the periosteum, is then dissected with the scalpel oriented toward the alveolar bone. This will ensure that the flap is not punctured.

The result from this sharp dissection is a very mobile flap that can easily be moved coronally. This mobility is achieved by carrying the dissection beyond the mucogingival junction. The papillae adjacent to the recession are then de-epithelialized with a new no. 15 blade and the flap sutured 0.5–1.0 mm coronal to the cemento-enamel junction. This is achieved using single interrupted sutures to secure the papilla areas and the vertical releasing inci-

sions (Fig. 8.4). The area is covered with a periodontal dressing and left to heal for 1 week. After 2 months (Fig. 8.5), the patient can start gently brushing the area.

SEMILUNAR CORONALLY POSITIONED FLAP

Technique

After proper local anesthesia, the recession is root planed thoroughly. With a no. 15 blade, a semilunar incision is made following the curvature of the free gingival margin that extends into the papillae (Fig. 8.6). One should avoid the papilla tips at this time (by at least 2 mm). Using a no. 15 blade or the Orban knife (Hu-Friedy, Chicago, IL, USA), insert the blade in the sulcus and connect to the apically made semilunar incision (Fig. 8.7). This is done through sharp dissection. You will then have a partial thickness flap that can be coronally pulled.

As always, when performing this type of procedure, it is important to keep the tip of the blade aimed at the alveolar bone while dissecting the flap; this prevents tissue perfora-

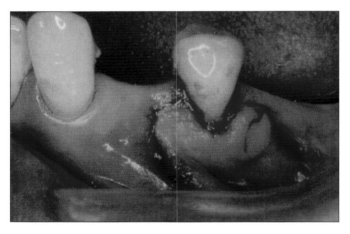

Figure 8.3. The partial thickness flap is elevated.

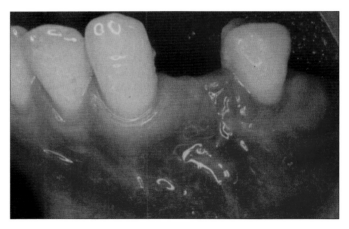

Figure 8.5. Healing after 2 months.

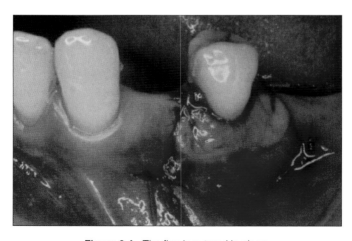

Figure 8.4. The flap is sutured in place.

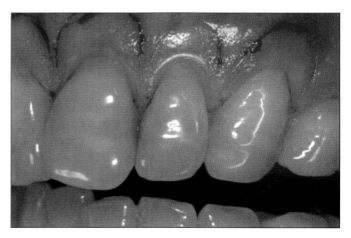

Figure 8.6. Semilunar incisions in the gingiva above the recessions affecting teeth 8–11.

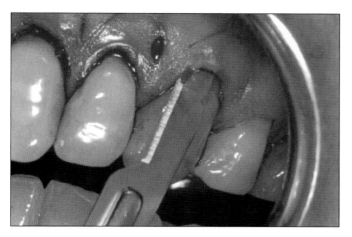

Figure 8.7. The blade inserted in the sulcus will connect the flap to the apical semilunar incisions.

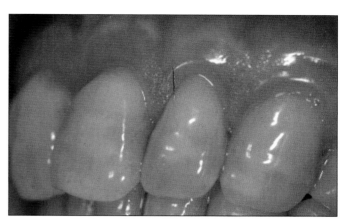

Figure 8.9. At 2 years after procedure, there is a slight marginal recession.

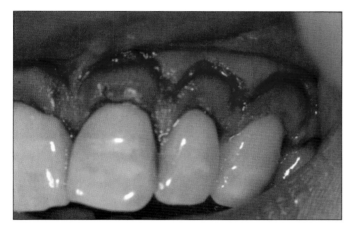

Figure 8.8. The semilunar flap is positioned coronally.

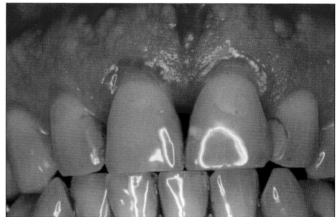

Figure 8.10. Teeth 8 and 9 have gingival recessions.

tion. The loosened flap, which is still connected at the papillae, is coronally repositioned to cover the recession (Fig. 8.8), held in place between fingers with light pressure, and covered with a periodontal dressing. No sutures are placed. The healing is uneventful (Fig. 8.9).

The advantages of this technique (Tarnow 1986) are (a) the flap lies passively on the recession after coronal positioning, (b) the vestibular depth stays the same, (c) the papillae stay intact, with no aesthetic compromise, and (d) suturing is not needed.

CORONALLY POSITIONED FLAP: ONE STAGE

Prerequisites

- Shallow marginal recession
- Minimum keratinized tissue width (3 mm)
- Periodontium not too thin

Technique

After proper local anesthesia, the teeth with the recession are root planed, and the root is treated with citric acid as described earlier (Fig. 8.10). A split-thickness flap with two vertical releasing incisions is raised, and the papillae are de-epithelialized (Figs. 8.11 & 8.12). The flap is coronally moved and secured to the de-epthelialized papillae with single interrupted sutures (5-0 silk or chromic gut) (Fig. 8.13). Pressure is applied, and a periodontal dressing is placed on the wound for 1 week. The healing is generally uneventful (Fig. 8.14).

Possible complications

The most common complication of a one-stage, coronally positioned flap is necrosis of the flap margins, which will occur if the partial thickness flap is too thin. This, in turn, could result in exposure of the underlying root surface and make an existing recession worse. Partial thickness flaps

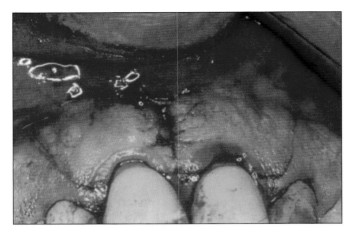

Figure 8.11. The labial frenum is eliminated, the wound sutured, and the flap design outlined.

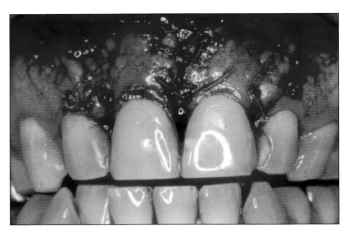

Figure 8.13. The flap is coronally moved and secured in place with 5-0 chromic gut, single interrupted sutures.

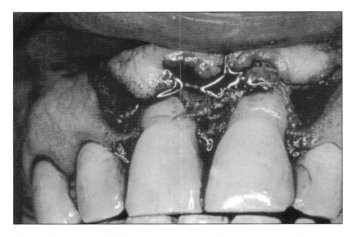

Figure 8.12. A partial thickness flap is elevated, and the papillae are de-epithelialized.

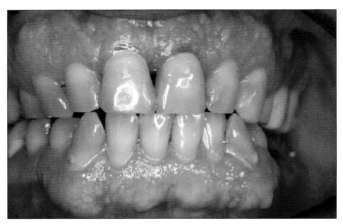

Figure 8.14. The area 1 year after the procedure.

are not indicated in areas of thin connective tissue (Wood et al. 1972). The gingival recession may also recur after a few years.

REFERENCES

Allen, E.P., & Miller, P.D. (1989) Coronal positioning of existing gingiva: Short term results in the treatment of shallow marginal tissue recession. *Journal of Periodontology* 60, 316–319.

Bernimoulin, J.P., Luscher, B., & Muhlemann, H. (1975) Coronally repositioned periodontal flap. *Journal of Clinical Periodontology* 2, 1–13.

Tarnow, D.P. (1986) Semilunar coronally repositioned flap. *Journal of Clinical Periodontology* 13, 182–185.

Wood, D.L., Hoag, F.M., Donnenfeld, O.W., & Rosenfeld, I.D. (1972) Alveolar crest reduction following full and partial thickness flaps. *Journal of Periodontology* 43, 141–144.

Chapter 9: Guided Tissue Regeneration

Serge Dibart

HISTORY

Guided tissue regeneration (GTR) is defined by the American Academy of Periodontology as a procedure attempting to regenerate lost periodontal structures through differential tissue responses (American Academy of Periodontology 1996). It involves the use of resorbable or nonresorbable barriers (membranes) to exclude epithelial and connective tissue cells from the root surface during wound healing. This is believed to facilitate the regeneration of lost cementum, periodontal ligament, and alveolar bone. In theory, this technique should result in reconstructing the attachment apparatus rather than just root coverage.

The membranes used during this procedure are most commonly made of materials such as expanded polytetrafluoroethylene (ePTFE), polyglactic acid, polylactic acid, and collagen. Pini-Prato et al. (1992) and Tinti & Vincenzi (1994) reported the use of an ePTFE membrane to treat gingival recessions. Cortellini et al. (1993) conducted a histological study on a patient, demonstrating that the root coverage obtained with the use of an ePTFE membrane, while treating a gingival recession, led to new connective tissue attachment and new bone formation. In 2001, Harris, while examining the histology of four teeth with gingival recessions treated with GTR, reported healing with a long junctional epithelium attachment without regeneration.

INDICATIONS

- Moderate to severe gingival recessions

- Thin palate

- Patient reluctant to have a second surgery site

ARMAMENTARIUM

This includes the basic surgical kit plus the following:

- Barrier membrane: resorbable (e.g., Resolut (W.L. Gore, Flagstaff, AZ, USA) XT, XTN2, or XTW1 and/or nonresorbable (e.g., Gore-Tex titanium reinforced TRN2, TRW2 or GTN1, GTN2, GTW1, or GTW2)

- Citric acid, pH 1 (40%), or 1 capsule of tetracycline hydrochloride (HCl), 250 mg

GUIDED TISSUE REGENERATION FOR ROOT COVERAGE

Technique

After proper anesthesia (Fig. 9.1), the recession is root planned thoroughly and flattened using a Gracey (Hu-Friedy, Chicago, IL, USA) curette or a back-action chisel (Fig. 9.2). The root is conditioned for 5 min with tetracycline paste. Two vertical releasing incisions are made at the line angles of the tooth with the recession (Fig. 9.3). These releasing incisions must pass the mucogingival junction for the flap to be mobile.

An intrasulcular incision connects the two verticals coronally. A full-thickness flap is raised using a periosteal elevator (24G) (Hu-Friedy) that will enable bone visibility 3 mm apical to the exposed root (Fig. 9.4). The flap is then converted to a partial thickness one apically that will enable coronal mobilization.

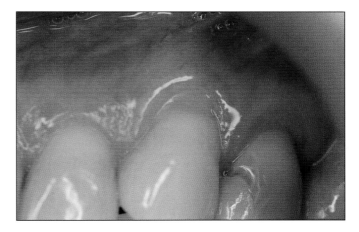

Figure 9.1. Tooth 11 with a moderate gingival recession.

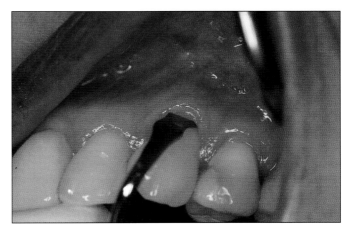

Figure 9.2. The exposed root surface is thoroughly scaled with a back-action chisel.

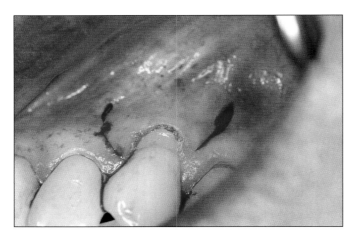

Figure 9.3. Two vertical incisions are placed, avoiding the interproximal papillae.

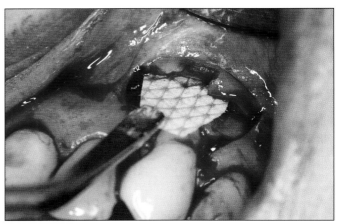

Figure 9.5. Trimming the reabsorbable membrane (Resolut) and adjusting it to fit the site.

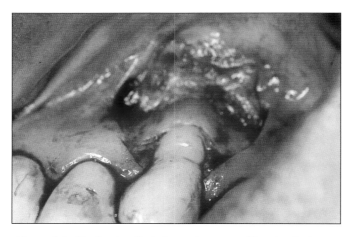

Figure 9.4. The flap is reflected exposing some of the alveolar bone.

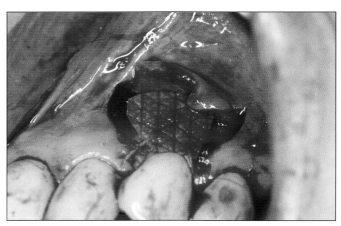

Figure 9.6. The membrane (Resolut) is secured in place with resorbable sutures.

At this stage, the buccal flap, full at the top and partial at the bottom, when moved coronally should be able to cover and lie passively on the recession. This is critical because any tension while suturing will affect the positive outcome of the procedure. The papillae are de-epithelialized, and the membrane is trimmed and adjusted to cover the recession (Fig. 9.5).

The membrane should extend approximately 2 mm beyond the borders of the recession mesially, distally, and apically. The membrane should be coronally placed at the level of the cemento-enamel junction and sutured in place with a circumferential suture and a palatally tied knot (Fig. 9.6).

The knot is then palatally tucked into the gingival sulcus. When the sulcus is shallow, a small intrasulcular incision

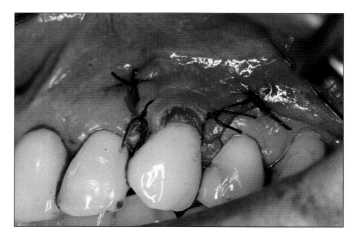

Figure 9.7. The buccal flap is sutured with the aim of covering as much of the membrane as possible.

will help deepen it. Once the membrane is secured, the buccal flap is coronally moved and secured to the papillae with interrupted sutures (Fig. 9.7). The releasing incisions are secured with single interrupted sutures, or with figure-eight sutures on both sides. It is important, whenever possible, to not leave the membrane exposed. To avoid this, the buccal flap is usually placed 0.5–1.0 mm coronal to the cemento-enamel junction to cover the underlying membrane.

A periodontal dressing is then applied on the wound and left for 1 week. It is advantageous to use a resorbable membrane with resorbable sutures when performing this procedure. Using a resorbable membrane with resorbable sutures eliminates the need for a second surgery, which usually follows 6 weeks later to remove the membrane. The area will heal uneventfully with predictable results as long as the flap was sutured tension free (Fig. 9.8).

Wound healing

Teflon/ePTFE membranes

These are nonresorbable, biocompatible membranes that require a second surgery for removal. There are two parts to this membrane. The first is an open microstructure collar inhibiting epithelial migration, and the second is an occlusive apron isolating the root surface from the surrounding tissues (Gottlow et al. 1986).

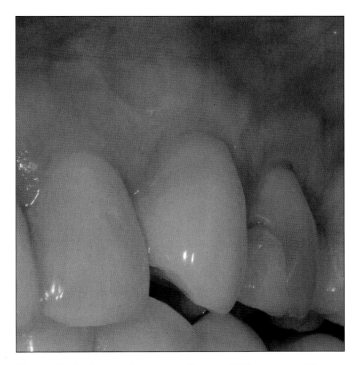

Figure 9.8. By 2 years after surgery, there is 100% coverage of the root surface.

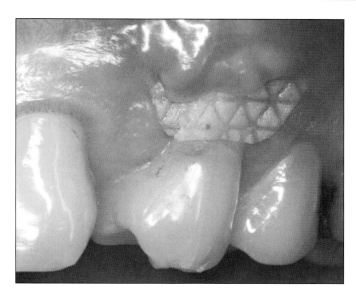

Figure 9.9. Membrane exposure 2 weeks after the surgery.

Polylactic acid membranes

These are biodegradable membranes degraded by hydrolysis. They do not require a second surgery for removal (Magnusson et al. 1988). The matrix barrier has an external layer and an internal layer separated by a space that will enable gingival connective tissue integration while excluding the epithelium (Gottlow et al. 1994).

The histology of one case (Cortellini et al. 1993) showed 3.66 mm of new connective tissue attachment, associated with 2.48 mm of new cementum and 1.84 mm of bone growth.

Possible complications

The most common complication is membrane exposure (Fig. 9.9). If the membrane is resorbable, and there are no signs of infection, the patient should be advised to rinse with chlorhexidine gluconate. With time, the membrane will disintegrate.

If the membrane is nonresorbable and the exposure limited, the patient is given a course of antibiotics (i.e., amoxicillin, 1.5 g/day for 7 days) and asked to rinse with chlorhexidine gluconate until removal of the membrane (after 6 weeks). An infected nonresorbable membrane should be removed (Nowzari et al. 1995).

Another complication is the perforation of the flap because of the inappropriate trimming of the membrane. This occurs if the membrane is stiff and the trimming has left sharp edges. It is important when trimming the membrane to have round angles to decrease the chances of flap perforation. If the membrane is exposed, treat it in the manner already outlined.

REFERENCES

American Academy of Periodontology (1996) *Annals of Periodontology World Workshop in Periodontics.* Chicago: American Academy of Periodontology, 1: 621.

Cortellini, P., Clauser, C., & Pini-Prato, G. (1993) Histologic assessment of new attachment following the treatment of a human buccal recession by means of a guided tissue regeneration procedure. *Journal of Periodontology* 64, 387–391.

Gottlow, J., Nyman, S., Lindhe, J., Karring, T., & Wennstrom, J. (1986) New attachment formation in the human periodontium by guided tissue regeneration: Case reports. *Journal of Clinical Periodontology* 13, 604–616.

Gottlow, J., Laurell, L., Lundgren, D., Mathisen, T., Nyman, S., Rylander, H., & Bogentoft, C. (1994) Periodontal tissue response to a new bioresorbable guided tissue regeneration device: A longitudinal study in monkeys. *International Journal of Periodontics and Restorative Dentistry* 14, 437–450.

Harris, R.J. (2001) Histologic evaluation of root coverage obtained with GTR in humans: A case report. *International Journal of Periodontics and Restorative Dentistry* 21, 240–251.

Magnusson, I., Batich, C., & Collins, B.R. (1988) New attachment formation following controlled tissue regeneration using biodegradable membranes. *Journal of Periodontology* 59, 1–6.

Nowzari, H., Matian, F., & Slots, J. (1995) Periodontal pathogens on polytetrafluoroethylene membrane for guided tissue regeneration inhibit healing. *Journal of Clinical Periodontology* 22, 469–474.

Pini-Prato, G., Tinti, C., Vincenzi, G., Magnani, C., Cortellini, P, & Clauser, C. (1992) Guided tissue regeneration versus mucogingival surgery in the treatment of human buccal gingival recession. *Journal of Periodontology* 63, 919–928.

Tinti, C., & Vincenzi, G.P. (1994) Expended polytetrafluoroethylene titanium reinforced membranes for regeneration of mucogingival recession defects: A 12-case report. *Journal of Periodontology* 65, 1088–1094.

Chapter 10: Acellular Dermal Matrix Graft (AlloDerm)

Serge Dibart

HISTORY

Acellular dermal matrix allograft, originally intended to cover burn wounds (Wainwright 1995), has been introduced as a less invasive alternative to soft tissue grafting (Silverstein & Callan 1997). This allograft is a freeze-dried, cell-free, dermal matrix comprised of a structurally integrated basement-membrane complex and extracellular matrix in which collagen bundles and elastic fibers are the main components (Wei et al. 2000).

INDICATIONS

- Soft tissue augmentation
- Multiple adjacent gingival recessions
- Lack of graftable palatal tissue
- Patient reluctant to have a second surgical site
- Correction of gingival/mucosal amalgam tattoos

ARMAMENTARIUM

This includes the basic surgical kit, AlloDerm, sterile saline, and two sterile dishes.

TECHNIQUE

After scaling and root planning, the root surfaces are conditioned. A partial thickness flap creating a pouch is formed using a no. 15 blade (Figs. 10.1 & 10.2). All these steps are similar to those described for the subepithelial connective tissue graft.

The AlloDerm is rehydrated in two consecutive 10- to 15-min sterile saline baths (depending on size and thickness of the piece used). The graft is inserted into the pouch with the connective tissue side—the bloody side—against the recipient bed. The papillae are de-epithelialized, and the graft is immobilized with resorbable sutures at the level of the cemento-enamel junction (Fig. 10.3). The buccal flap is then sutured over the AlloDerm to cover the graft as much as possible. It is important to not leave any AlloDerm exposed, if possible (Fig. 10.4).

POSTOPERATIVE INSTRUCTIONS

Postoperative instructions include systemic antibiotherapy for 7 days after the surgery. This is helpful to avoid complications. Nonsteroidal or steroidal anti-inflammatory drugs should be prescribed to keep the pain and swelling down (Greenwell et al. 2004).

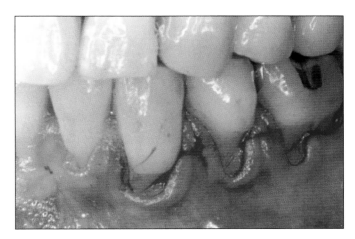

Figure 10.1. Envelope incision: a pouch is created.

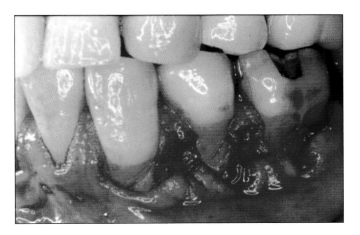

Figure 10.2. The roots are scaled, and the pouch is ready to accommodate the graft.

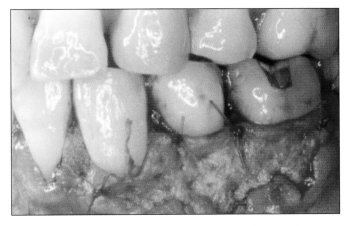

Figure 10.3. The AlloDerm is trimmed to fit the pouch, cover the roots, and suture to the papillae. These have been de-epithelialized.

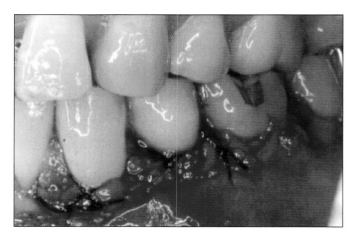

Figure 10.4. The buccal flap is sutured over the AlloDerm by using a sling suture to provide the graft with maximum coverage; 100% coverage is ideal.

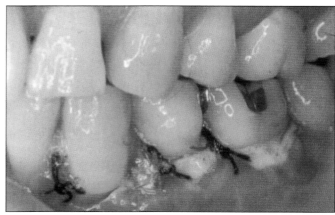

Figure 10.5. By 1 week after surgery, some of the AlloDerm is exposed. The whitishness is a normal feature of this healing process.

GRAFT HEALING

Significant revascularization occurs in just over 1 week. AlloDerm is repopulated with cells and will begin remodeling into the patient's own tissue over the next 3–6 months. Up to 41% shrinkage of the graft has been reported during that period (Batista et al. 2001). The material will also take the characteristics of the underlying and surrounding tissues (for example, keratinized tissue or mucosa). Do not be concerned by the whitishness of the graft after surgery; it is not tissue necrosis. This color reflects normal healing (Fig. 10.5).

The final results are seen 2–3 years later (Fig. 10.6), sometimes with the help of a creeping attachment. It is important to remember that, when evaluating the results, the concept of gain of attached gingiva or keratinized gingiva is replaced by gain of gingival volume. The absence of keratinized tissue with this technique after successful root coverage is not uncommon, nor detrimental to the results.

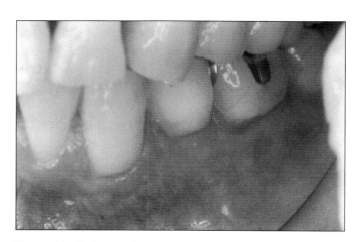

Figure 10.6. By 3 years after surgery, the recessions have been covered.

REMOVAL AND CORRECTION OF AMALGAM TATTOO

The tattooed area is excised and the recipient bed prepared, as though for a free gingival graft procedure. The possible remnants of embedded amalgam particles are carefully removed from the underlying tissues, and one piece of AlloDerm is cut to size and adapted to the site. The AlloDerm is sutured carefully to the gingival margins, and a few crisscross sutures are added to immobilize the AlloDerm and prevent exfoliation. The area is then covered with a periodontal dressing (Figs. 10.7–10.10).

GINGIVAL GRAFTING TO INCREASE SOFT TISSUE VOLUME

For gingival grafting to increase soft tissue volume, apply the aforementioned technique, with the exception of the

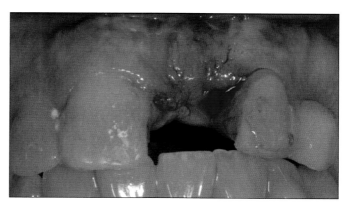

Figure 10.7. Amalgam tattoo on the gingiva, in the aesthetic zone.

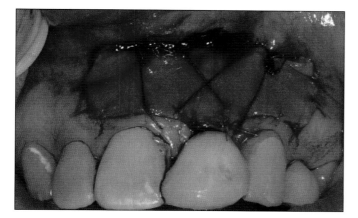

Figure 10.8. Amalgam tattoo excised and AlloDerm grafted and sutured.

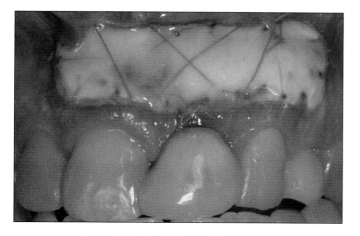

Figure 10.9. Results 1 week after surgery.

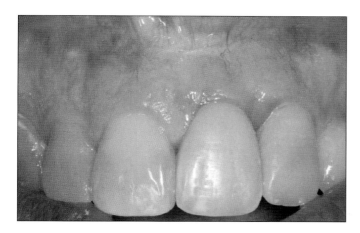

Figure 10.10. Results 1 year after surgery. The mucogingival problem has been corrected and the final prosthesis inserted.

bed (prepared directly below the mucogingival junction) (Figs. 10.11–10.13). Shrinkage of the graft is inevitable, so plan accordingly.

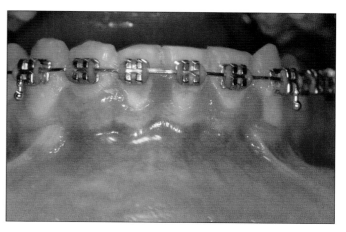

Figure 10.11. Thin gingival biotype requiring soft tissue augmentation in conjunction with orthodontic treatment.

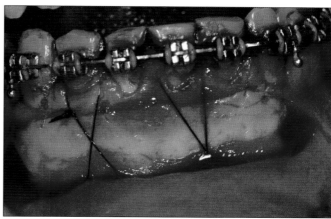

Figure 10.12. AlloDerm sutured in place.

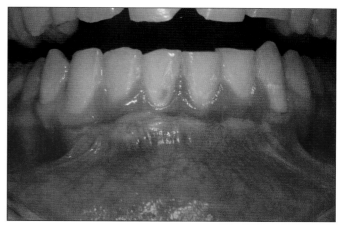

Figure 10.13. Healing of the graft at 1 year.

POSSIBLE COMPLICATIONS

A possible complication of the procedure is the exfoliation of the AlloDerm if it is not well secured. AlloDerm tends to swell during the week after surgery. Another complication is infection of the graft, necessitating its removal. Having the patient take antibiotics the day before surgery can prevent this. The patient can also be given anti-inflammatory drugs (steroidal and nonsteroidal) to control postoperative swelling and pain (Greenwell and al. 2004). This is particularly useful when using AlloDerm in ridge augmentation in edentulous areas (see Chapter 12).

REFERENCES

Batista, E.L., Batista, F.C., & Novaes, A.B. (2001) Management of soft tissue ridge deformities with acellular dermal matrix: Clinical approach and outcome after 6 months of treatment [Case series]. *Journal of Periodontology* 72(2), 265–273.

Greenwell, H., Vance, G., Munninger, B., & Johnston, H. (2004) Superficial-layer split-thickness flap for maximal flap release and coronal positioning: A surgical technique. *International Journal of Periodontics and Restorative Dentistry* 24, 521–527.

Silverstein, L.H., & Callan, D.P. (1997) An acellular dermal matrix allograft substitute for palatal donor tissue. *Postgraduate Dentistry* 3, 14–21.

Wainwright, D.J. (1995) Use of an acellular allograft dermal matrix (AlloDerm) in the management of full-thickness burns. *Burns* 21, 243–248.

Wei, P.C., Laurell, L., Geivelis, M., Lingen, M.W., & Maddalozzo, D. (2000) Acellular dermal matrix allografts to achieve increased attached gingiva. Part 1. A clinical study. *Journal of Periodontology* 71, 1297–1305.

Chapter 11: Labial Frenectomy Alone or in Combination with a Free Gingival Autograft

Serge Dibart and Mamdouh Karima

HISTORY

Frena, which are triangle-shaped folds found in the maxillary and mandibular alveolar mucosa, are located between the central incisors and canine premolar area. Frena may be long and thin, or short and broad. Labial frenum attachments have been described as mucosal, gingival, papillary, and papilla penetrating (Placek et al. 1974a & b).

Insertion points of the frena may become a problem when the gingival margin is involved (Corn 1964). This may be the result of an unusually high insertion of the frenum or marginal recession of the gingiva. High frenal insertion can distend and pull the marginal gingiva or papilla away from the tooth when the lip is stretched. This condition may be conducive to plaque accumulation and inhibit proper oral hygiene.

Aberrant frena can be treated by frenectomy or frenotomy procedures. The terms *frenectomy* and *frenotomy* signify operations that differ in degree of surgical approach. *Frenectomy* is a complete removal of the frenum, including its attachment to the underlying bone, and may be required for correction of abnormal diastema between maxillary central incisors (Friedman 1957). *Frenotomy* is the incision and relocation of the frenal attachment.

Abnormal frenal attachments occur most often on the facial surface between the maxillary and mandibular central incisors and in the canine and premolar areas (Whinston 1956). High frenal attachments on the lingual surface are less common. Orthodontic closure of diastema without excision of the associated frena are clinically associated with relapse separation of the teeth (Edwards 1977).

A frenectomy is a simple surgical procedure that can be performed separately (that is, for orthodontic reasons) or in conjunction with a free gingival graft (that is, to treat a gingival recession, increase the amount of attached gingival, or deepen the vestibule).

INDICATIONS

- Eliminate tension on the gingival margin (frenum-pull concomitant with or without gingival recession)
- Facilitate orthodontic treatment
- Facilitate home care

ARMAMENTARIUM

This includes the basic kit plus a mosquito hemostat.

TECHNIQUE

Surgical steps for frenum removal

Grasp the frenum (Fig. 11.1) with a slightly curved hemostat inserted into the depth of the vestibule. Incise along the upper surface of the hemostat, extending beyond the tip. Make a similar incision along the undersurface of the hemostat until the hemostat is free.

Remove the triangular resected portion of the frenum with the hemostat. This exposes the underlying brushlike fibrous attachment to the bone (Fig. 11.2). Use the curved scissor to remove any dense fibers from the wound. Extend the lip and determine whether there is still pull on the periosteum. Clean the field of operation and pack it with wet gauze until bleeding subsides.

Suturing technique

Suture the edges of the diamond-shaped wound together by using 5-0 silk in simple interrupted fashion (Fig. 11.3). Place three sutures across the wound margin to reduce postoperative discomfort and promote healing. Then apply the periodontal dressing to protect the surgical field.

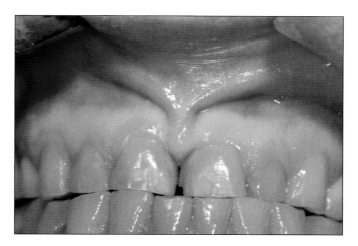

Figure 11.1. Maxillary labial frenum before frenectomy.

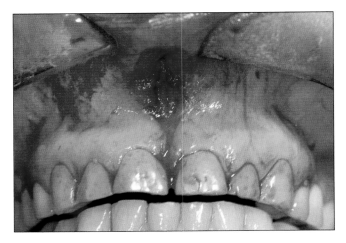

Figure 11.2. Excision of the maxillary frenum.

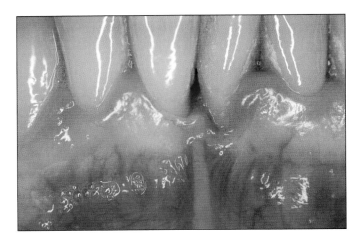

Figure 11.4. Another case of free gingival graft used to cover a buccal recession on tooth 24.

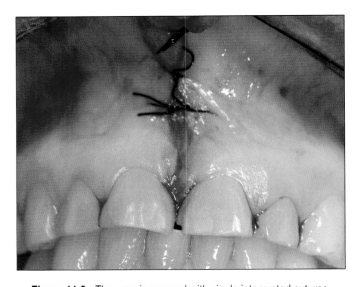

Figure 11.3. The area is secured with single interrupted sutures.

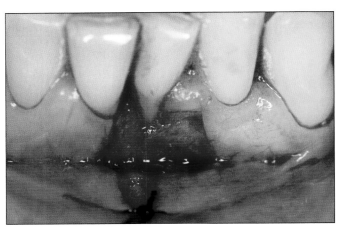

Figure 11.5. The recipient bed has been prepared, and the labial frenum excised to accommodate the gingival autograft.

POSSIBLE COMPLICATIONS

Frenectomy may result in scar formation that could prevent the mesial movement of the central incisors (West 1968). However, frenectomy is typically a safe surgical procedure with no notable complications.

LABIAL FRENECTOMY IN ASSOCIATION WITH A FREE GINGIVAL AUTOGRAFT

See Figs. 11.4–11.8.

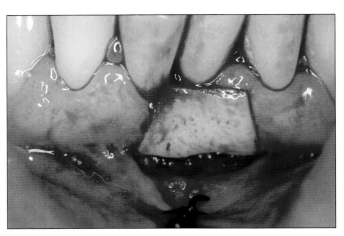

Figure 11.6. The free gingival graft is in place, with the connective tissue side against the recipient bed.

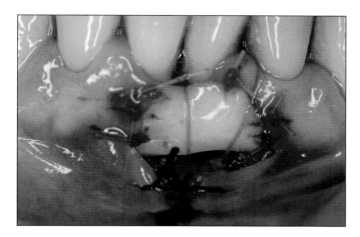

Figure 11.7. The graft is secured with resorbable 5-0 gut sutures.

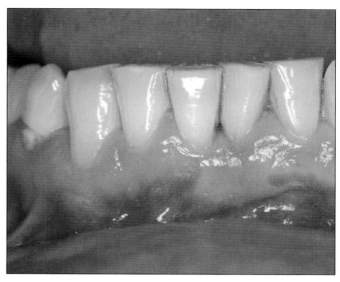

Figure 11.8. The area 1 year after surgery. Root coverage has been achieved, the amount of keratinized tissue has increased, and the frenum has been excised. Notice the restoration of the mesial papilla of tooth 24.

REFERENCES

Corn, H. (1964) Edentulous area pedicle grafts in mucogingival surgery. *Periodontics* 2, 229–242.

Edwards, J.G. (1977) The diastema, the frenum, the frenectomy: A clinical study. *American Journal of Orthodontics* 71, 489–508.

Friedman, N. (1957) Mucogingival surgery. *Texas Dental Journal* 75, 358–362.

Placek, M., Skach, M., & Mrklas, L. (1974a) Problems with the lip frenulum in periodontics. I. Classification and epidemiology of tendons of the lip frenulum. *Ceskoslovenska Stomatologie* 74, 385–391.

Placek, M., Skach, M., & Mrklas, L. (1974b) Problems of the labial frenum attachment in periodontics. II. Attempts to determine the resistance of periodontium to the influence of individual types of the labial frenum attachment. *Ceskoslovenska Stomatologie* 74, 401–406.

West, E. (1968) Diastema: A cause for concern. *Dental Clinics of North America* 425–434.

Whinston, G.J. (1956) Frenetomy and mucobuccal fold resection used in periodontal therapy. *New York Dental Journal* 22, 495–497.

Chapter 12: Preprosthetic Ridge Augmentation: Hard and Soft

Serge Dibart and Luigi Montesani

HISTORY

In 1983, Seibert (1983a, 1983b) classified the different types of alveolar ridge defects that a clinician may encounter while planning a prosthetic rehabilitation. His classification described the following three clinical situations:

- Class I alveolar ridge defects have a horizontal loss of tissue with normal ridge height.

- Class II alveolar ridge defects have a vertical loss of tissue with normal ridge width.

- Class III alveolar ridge defects have a combination of class I and class II resulting in loss of normal height and width.

The reconstruction of a normal alveolar housing, in height and width, is imperative to achieve a harmonious balance between biology, function, and aesthetics.

INDICATIONS

The indications of alveolar ridge defects occur when the loss of substance compromises the positive outcome of a prosthetic restoration. This is particularly true in the aesthetic zone, and most of the time is caused by periodontal disease, careless tooth extraction, chronic infection, implant failure, congenital diseases, trauma, or neoplasm.

The loss of gingiva or bone can be detrimental to the successful placement of an implant or a fixed partial denture. This loss of substance can be avoided by socket preservation or immediate implant placement, or treated with soft and hard tissue grafting.

When planning treatment for corrective surgery, it is important to inform the patient that a single procedure may not repair the defect, so a second, or sometimes even a third, procedure is sometimes warranted. A Seibert class I defect is easier to treat than a class II, which, in turn, is easier to treat than a class III. A class III defect will require

multiple grafting. In addition, the prognosis is better in the case of horizontal defects as opposed to vertical or combined defects.

These defects can be corrected by the following procedures (Table 12.1).

Soft tissue grafts

These are the roll technique (small to moderate class I defects), free gingival onlay grafts (class I, II, and III defects), connective tissue inlay grafts (class I defects), wedge-sandwich grafts (class I and small class II), and soft tissue allografts [AlloDerm (acellular dermal matrix allograft); LifeCell, Branchburg, NJ, USA] for class I, II and III.

Hard Tissue Grafts

These are guided bone regeneration (GBR) with autogenous bone grafts, bone allografts, bone xenografts, synthetic bone substitutes, and block grafts.

Combination of soft and hard tissue grafts

The hard tissue graft used will depend on the extent and severity of the defect and on the type of prosthetic restoration that will follow. When an implant-supported fixed prosthesis is planned, a bone graft is needed with or without a soft tissue graft. However, when a fixed partial denture is planned, a soft tissue graft could be sufficient. It is important to keep in mind that a patient may need more than one surgery to correct a defect. In certain specific cases, procedures such as edentulous ridge expansion (ERE), distraction osteogenesis, and orthodontic treatment can be performed in conjunction with or in lieu of grafting.

ARMAMENTARIUM

This includes a basic surgical kit plus the following:

- Polytetrafluoroethylene sutures [Gore-Tex (W.L.Gore, Flagstaff, AZ, USA), suture CV-5]

TABLE 12.1. Soft tissue versus hard tissue augmentation

Soft tissue grafting	Hard tissue grafting
Mild to moderate defects (3mm–6mm)	Moderate to severe defects (> 4mm)
Horizontal defects	Horizontal and vertical defects
Fixed partial denture	Implant therapy
Availability of soft tissue	Inadequate soft tissue quantity
Questionable long–term stability	Stable with time
May need multiple augmentations	

Adapted from Pini-Prato et al. (2004).

- Barrier membranes: resorbable [i.e., Resolut (W.L. Gore), Bio-Gide (Osteohealth, Shirley, NY, USA), or Ossix (3i, Palm Beach Gardens, FL, USA)] and nonresorbable [i.e., Gore-Tex expanded polytetrafluoroethylene (e-PTFE)]

- Bone allograft or substitute [i.e., Regenaform (Exactech, Gainesville, FL, USA), Dembone (Pacific Coast Tissue Bank, Los Angeles, CA, USA), Bio-Oss (Osteohealth), or Cerasorb (Curasan, Research Triangle Park, NC, USA)]

- Acellular Dermal Matrix: AlloDerm (LifeCell)

- Fixation screws: OsteoMed (Dallas, TX, USA)

- Collagen plugs: CollaPlug (Zimmer, Warsaw, IN, USA)

- Purified *n*-butyl cyanoacrylate glue (PeriAcryl) (GluStitch; Delta, BC, Canada)

SOFT TISSUE GRAFT

Technique

The soft tissue graft technique is particularly well suited when a fixed partial denture restoration is planned (Figs. 12.1 & 12.2). After proper anesthesia has been established, a partial thickness flap is elevated (Fig. 12.3). The horizontal crestal incision is slightly palatal or lingual with two vertical releasing incisions when necessary. Whenever possible, the vertical releasing incisions should be away from the external borders of the anticipated graft.

The partial thickness flap is raised and dissected beyond the mucogingival line to achieve coronal mobility. A connective tissue graft is harvested from the palate (Figs. 12.4 & 12.5), or a piece of AlloDerm is used when there is not enough autogenous tissue available. This graft is inserted under the buccal flap (Fig. 12.6) and secured to the periosteum with resorbable sutures (5-0 chromic gut P-3 needle).

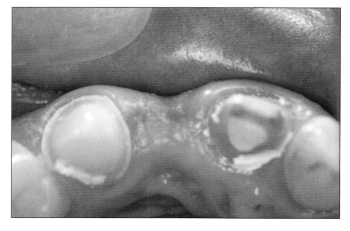

Figure 12.2. Occlusal view without the temporary restoration.

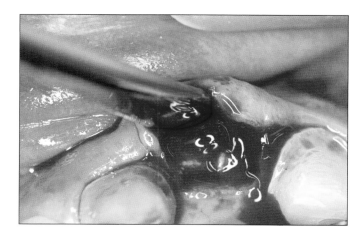

Figure 12.3. The horizontal incision is made and continued intrasulcularly to teeth 9 and 11. This helps with the sharp dissection and mobilizes the flap. An alternative would be to put two vertical incisions on each side of the area to be augmented.

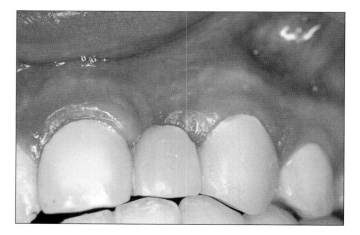

Figure 12.1. Seibert class I defect. The gingival buccal concavity needs to be augmented for a better aesthetic outcome. The restoration planned here is a fixed partial denture; hence the need for a soft tissue graft only.

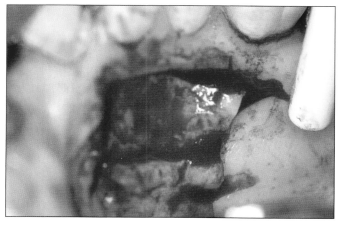

Figure 12.4. A trapdoor is opened in the palate to harvest the connective tissue graft to be used to correct the defect.

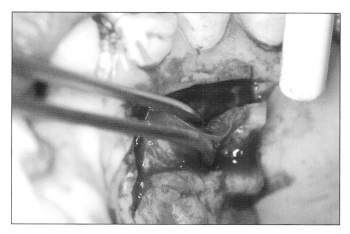

Figure 12.5. The harvest of the piece of connective tissue. The desired length and thickness have been determined by the size and shape of the defect to be corrected.

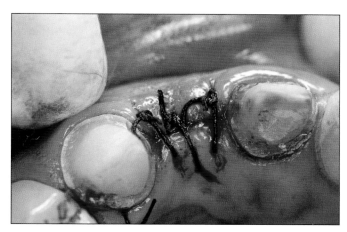

Figure 12.7. Once the connective tissue graft has been secured, the flaps are secured using single interrupted sutures.

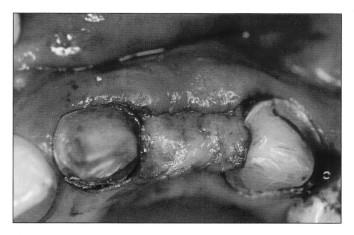

Figure 12.6. The graft is inserted and positioned into the wound. It will be secured to the periosteum bucally with an intraperiosteal horizontal mattress resorbable suture.

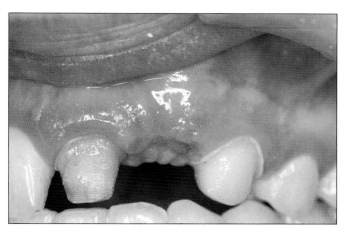

Figure 12.8. Buccal view of the augmented site 2 weeks after the surgery.

The partial thickness flap is then mobilized and coronally pulled to cover the graft. Single interrupted sutures are used to close the wound by primary intention (Fig. 12.7). It is advisable to keep the sutures in place for 2 weeks to ensure enough healing of the site (Figs. 12.8–12.10).

CLINICAL CROWN REDUCTION USING A CONNECTIVE TISSUE GRAFT

Use this technique when the crown preparation extends too far apically with or without a lack of attached gingiva (Figs. 12.11–12.20).

HARD TISSUE GRAFT

Hard tissue grafts are primarily used when an implant-supported restoration is planned. The hard tissue augmentation can be done with block grafts (autografts and allografts), particulate grafts (cortical and cancellous),

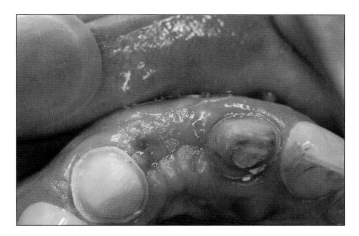

Figure 12.9. Occlusal view of the augmented site 2 weeks after the surgery. The buccal curvature has been restored.

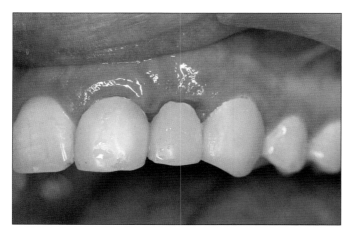

Figure 12.10. The pontic of the temporary bridge has been modified to apply light positive pressure to the area. This will help simulate papilla presence on each side of the final restoration (tooth 10).

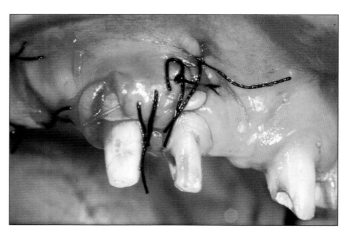

Figure 12.13. A connective tissue graft is inserted under a coronally positioned flap and secured using resorbable and silk sutures. The graft is placed on the freshly prepared root surface to re-create a zone of attached gingiva and modify the clinical crown length.

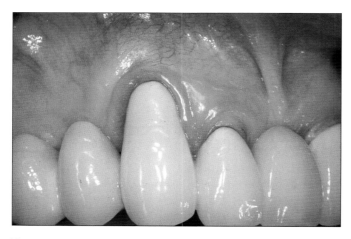

Figure 12.11. Unpleasant aesthetics as a result of iatrogenic dentistry (inadequate position of the crown margin and tooth preparation) requiring a correction of tooth 6. There is a gingival roll and inflammation around the maxillary canine and an inadequate amount of attached gingiva.

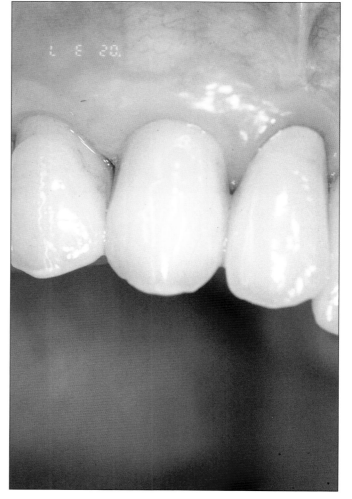

Figure 12.14. Final restoration 1 year later. A band of attached gingiva has been established, and pleasing aesthetics have resulted from the new position of the crown margin (tooth 6).

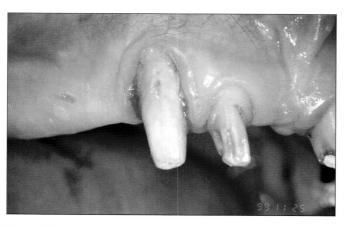

Figure 12.12. Removal of the old fixed prosthetic restoration and flattening of the exposed root and margin (rotary and hand instrumentation) in preparation for the connective tissue graft.

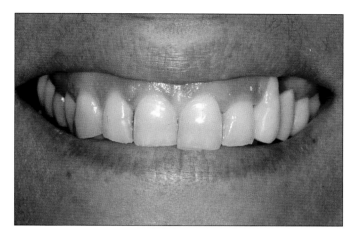

Figure 12.15. Unpleasant smile due to uneven marginal tissue height and loss of gingival volume (teeth 11 and 12).

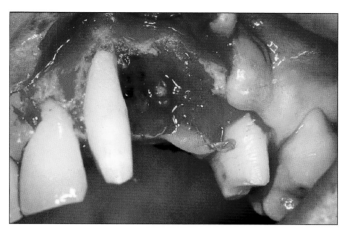

Figure 12.17. Extraction of tooth 12 and root preparation of tooth 11. Degranulation of the extraction site and preparation of the recipient bed.

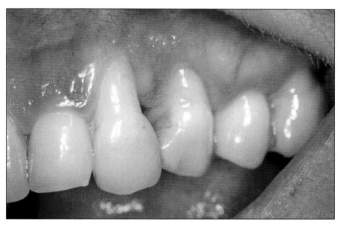

(a)

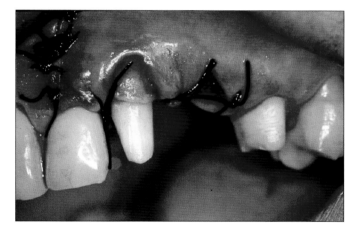

Figure 12.18. A connective tissue graft extending from tooth 10 to tooth 13 is inserted to correct the existing gingival recession on tooth 11, reestablishing a normal buccal-lingual ridge dimension.

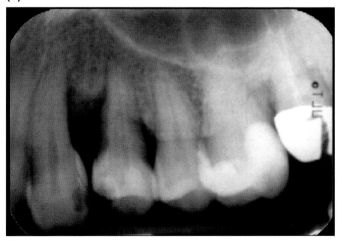

(b)

Figure 12.16. a: Miller class III with localized severe chronic periodontitis affecting teeth 11 and 12. **b:** Periapical radiograph of teeth 11 and 12.

xenografts, or synthetic materials. The use of a barrier membrane is recommended with the placement of a bone graft to minimize resorption and enhance the outcome of the procedure (Antoun et al. 2001; Von Arx et al. 2001).

The choice of materials is usually dictated by the existing anatomy, the patient's medical history, and the size of the defect. Autogenous bone grafts, the osteogenic gold standard, have limitations, such as availability, morbidity, risk of vascular and neurological injury, and increased surgical time.

Osteoinductive allografts and osteoconductive allografts, on the other hand, are available in unlimited quantity, do not necessitate a second surgical site, have a decreased rate of patient morbidity, and shorten the time of the surgical procedure. One of their major drawbacks is the potential risk of disease transmission (Moore et al. 2001).

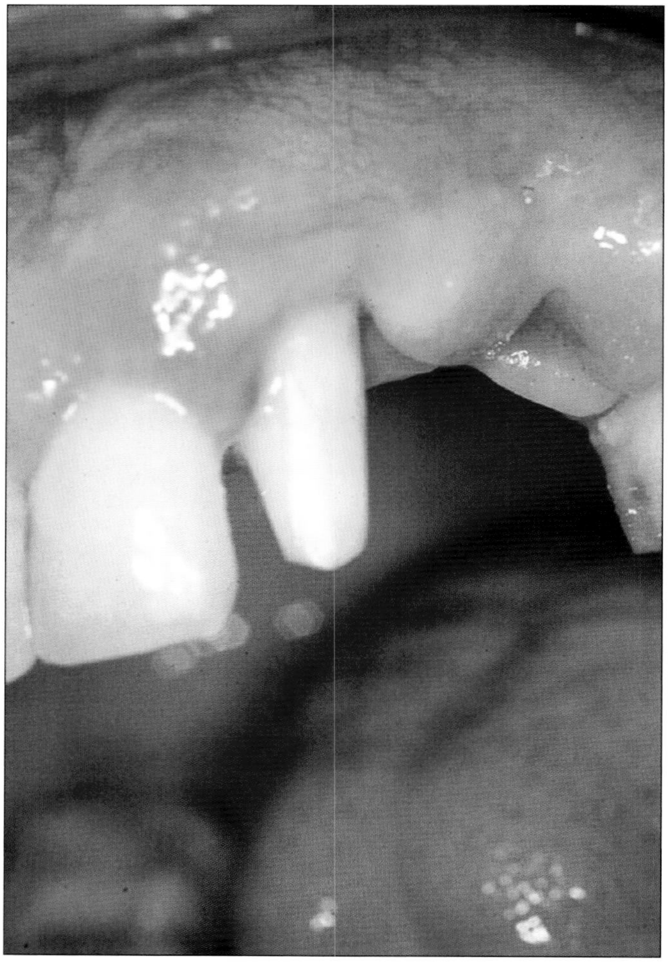

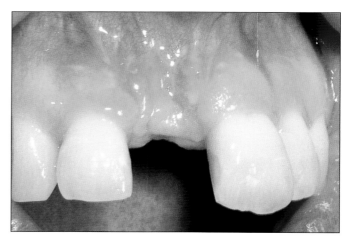

Figure 12.19. Healing at 2 months. An interdental papilla has been created by the judicious use of the temporary prosthesis (soft tissue conditioning).

COMBINATION GRAFTS: HARD AND SOFT TISSUES

This is used to correct an important defect affecting the alveolar bone and soft tissue volumes (Figs. 12.21–12.39)

EDENTULOUS RIDGE EXPANSION

Also known as ridge splitting, this technique is useful when there is a narrow crest, which is wider apically, with enough bone height but less than 5 mm of crestal bone width, and you plan an implant-supported prosthesis. The bone at the crest should not be all cortical, because it will make this technique difficult.

The purpose of the procedure is to reposition the buccal cortical plate and increase the alveolar width by expending the edentulous ridge. In 1990, Scipioni & Bruschi introduced

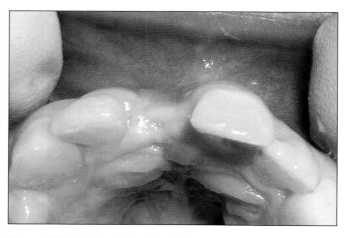

Figure 12.21. Seibert class I defect. The restoration planned here is an implant-supported crown; hence the bone tissue graft planned.

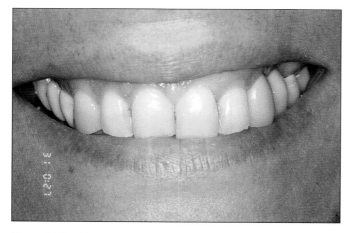

Figure 12.20. Healing at 1 year. The result is acceptable, aesthetics have improved, and the patient is satisfied.

Figure 12.22. Occlusal view of the defect showing the buccal concavity that will be augmented with a bone graft.

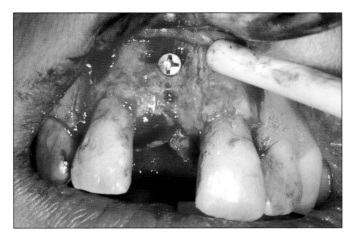

Figure 12.23. A full-thickness flap has been elevated, with a horizontal incision that is slightly palatal to the midcrest and two vertical releasing incisions. A 10-mm OsteoMed screw has been inserted halfway through the alveolar bone. This screw will serve as an anchor to the bone allograft (Regenaform) that will be placed next. The area receiving the graft has been decorticated by using a small round carbide burr.

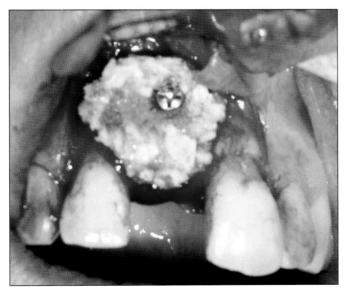

Figure 12.24. The Regenaform-block graft (10 × 10 × 5 mm), once softened, has been pushed through the screw and molded to fit the defect. When the defect is large, a second screw and a bigger graft may be necessary.

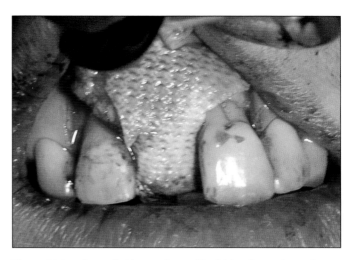

Figure 12.25. A resorbable membrane (Ossix) has been trimmed to the appropriate size and placed over the bone graft. The membrane is tucked under the palatal flap before suturing. The buccal flap is to be undermined to achieve coverage of the membrane and graft passively.

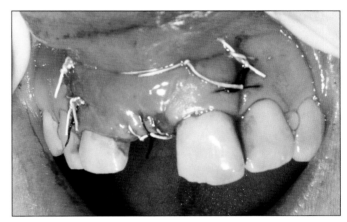

Figure 12.26. A horizontal mattress buccally and palatally with a Gore-Tex suture will hold the flaps up without tension and keep the membrane down on the bone. Additional single interrupted sutures will close the wound by primary intention.

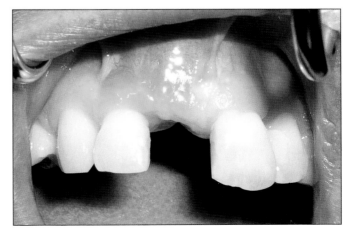

Figure 12.27. The area 1 year later. Buccal view.

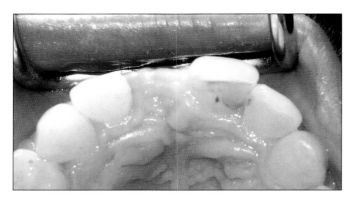

Figure 12.28. The area 1 year later. Occlusal view.

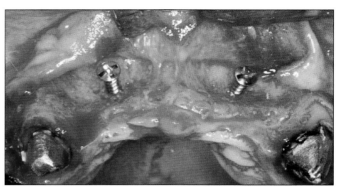

Figure 12.31. Two OsteoMed screws (1.6 × 10 mm) placed halfway into the alveolar bone.

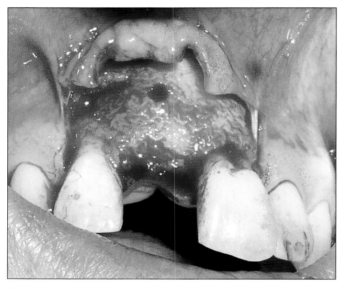

Figure 12.29. The area 1 year later at reentry and implant placement. The fixation screw was once where the red dot is.

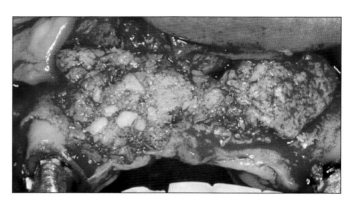

Figure 12.32. Two blocks of Regenaform (10 × 10 × 5 mm) molded and placed on the OsteoMed screws.

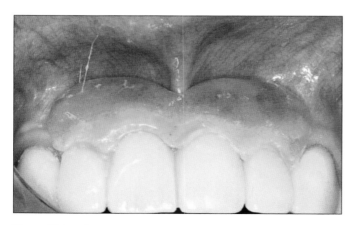

Figure 12.30. Severe vestibular and occlusal defect filled with an acrylic prosthesis to provide lip support.

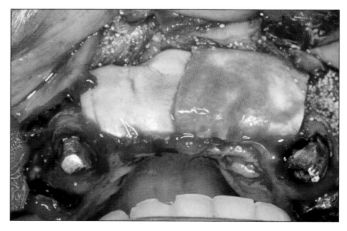

Figure 12.33. AlloDerm is used as a membrane to protect the bone graft and as a soft tissue graft to build up the vestibule. The AlloDerm is tucked under the palatal flap and secured coronally and apically to the periosteum by using resorbable sutures.

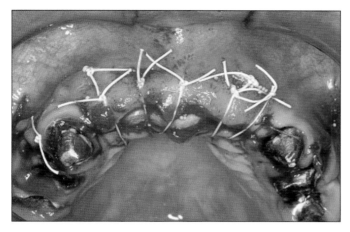

Figure 12.34. The buccal flap is coronally advanced by releasing the flap apically and secured by using horizontal mattress and single interrupted sutures (Gore-Tex). Some of the AlloDerm is left exposed, which allows for minimal coronal advancement of the flap and maintenance of the original vestibular depth.

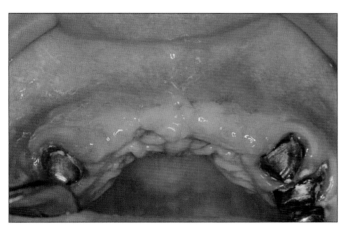

Figure 12.35. The area 3 months after the procedure.

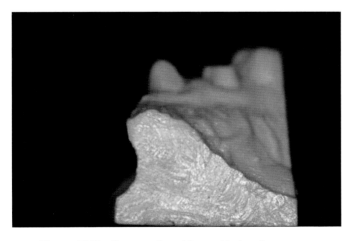

Figure 12.36. Cross section of the cast before the surgery.

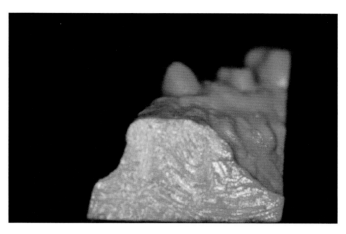

Figure 12.37. Cross section of the cast after the surgery. Notice the amount of tissue volume gained.

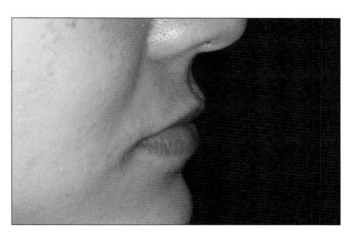

Figure 12.38. The patient's profile before the surgery. Notice the concavity of the upper lip due to the vestibular hard and soft tissue defect.

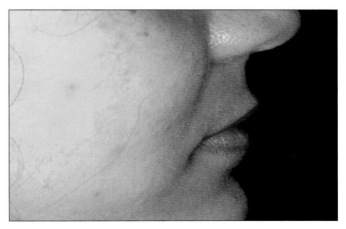

Figure 12.39. The patient's profile 3 months after surgery. Support has been provided to the upper lip, making for a better aesthetic profile.

the bony flap in conjunction with hand chisels to expand the alveolar ridge further (Scipioni et al. 1994, 1999). In 1994, Summers introduced a ridge-expansion technique using hand osteotomes. With the right indication, this procedure enables a surgeon to place an implant in a Seibert class I defect in one session, without the need of a bone graft.

Technique

Step-by-step illustration of the ridge splitting/expansion technique allowing the placement of an implant in a Seibert class I anterior ridge defect (Figs. 12.40–12.51)

SOCKET PRESERVATION

Sometimes it is necessary to extract teeth for reasons such as root fracture, periapical pathology, extensive decay, or periodontal disease. Careful removal of the tooth is completed atraumatically by using periotomes and gentle rotation movements with the forceps. Vertical and horizontal bone resorption is an inevitable natural phenomenon; there is 40% of bone height and 60% of bone width lost at 6 months (Lekovic et al. 1997, 1998).

This is further compounded by the location of the tooth to be extracted and the biotype of the patient, such as thin versus thick biotype, the former being a disadvantage. The anterior maxilla area is particularly at risk because the bone plates are thin and subject to resorption at the time of tooth removal. This can lead to the loss of bone contour

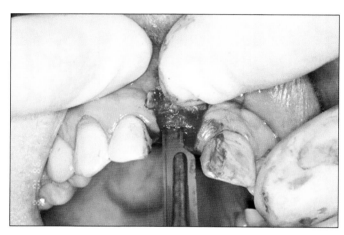

Figure 12.42. A conservative full-thickness buccal flap is raised to expose the crestal bone. Two vertical releasing incisions are placed to help mobilize the flap coronally at the end of the procedure (the flap is full thickness at the top and partial thickness at the bottom). The splitting of the ridge is initiated by using a no. 15 blade that is gently hammered in for about 5 mm.

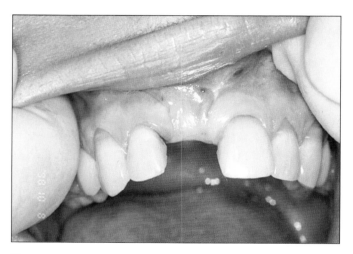

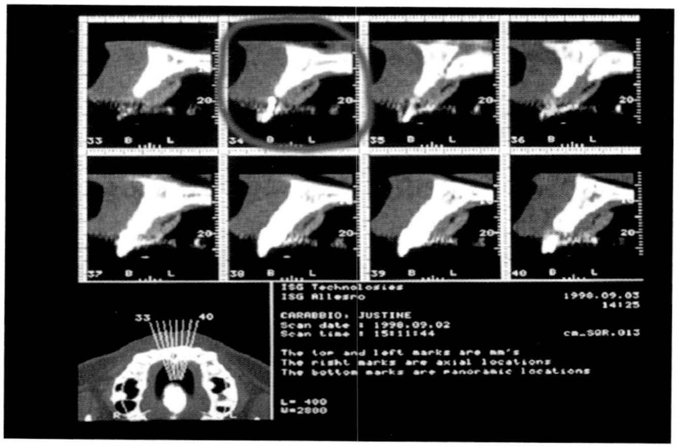

Figure 12.40. Tooth 8 is missing and will be replaced by an implant-supported crown to restore aesthetics and function.

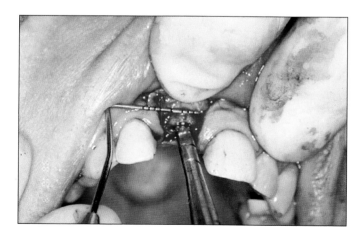

Figure 12.43. The splitting of the ridge is continued by using a bibevel osteotome chisel that will go slightly deeper than the blade and will expand the ridge to the buccal. Do not to create a single large fracture. Note the minimal flap reflection.

Figure 12.41. A computed-tomographic scan of the area shows a crestal bony width incompatible with successful implant placement.

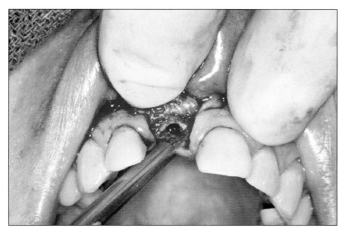

Figure 12.44. Once the midcrestal groove has been created and adequate depth obtained, the osteotomy is performed to the desired length with a 2.0-mm twist drill. This is often followed by the use of expanding osteotomes, which will condense the bone as they are expanding the osteotomy site, or proceeding with the next 3.0-mm drill.

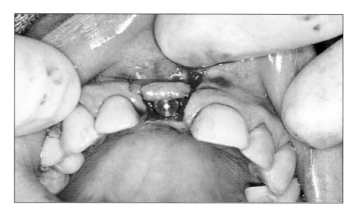

Figure 12.47. The blue mount has been removed and the cover screw tightened in place.

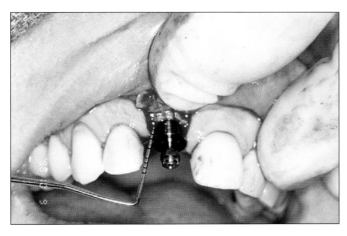

Figure 12.45. The implant is inserted carefully.

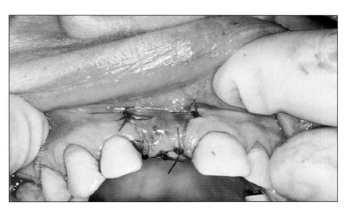

Figure 12.48. The flap is now gently advanced coronally by releasing it from the underlying periosteum (split-thickness flap) and sutured by primary intention with single interrupted sutures.

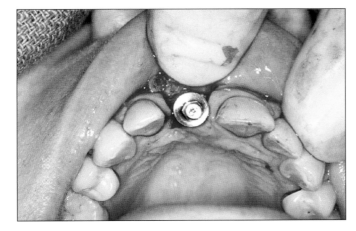

Figure 12.46. Occlusal view showing the satisfactory placement of the implant in the maxillary arch.

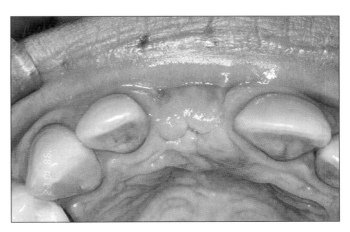

Figure 12.49. Occlusal view of the area 4 months after surgery.

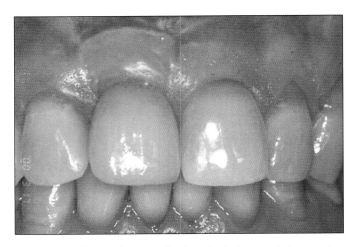

Figure 12.50. Tooth 8 is restored with an implant-supported crown. A gingival graft was needed because of gingival scars from multiple endodontic procedures.

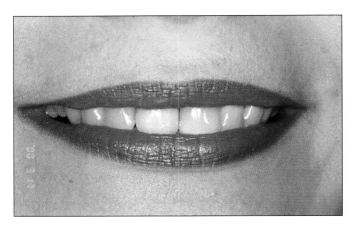

Figure 12.51. The patient's smile at the time of crown insertion.

and poor aesthetics. To avoid this, socket preservation becomes necessary at the time of extraction.

The Bio-Col (Bio-Oss + Collaplug) technique (Sclar 2003) or its modification helps minimize the amount of bone loss and preserve ridge aesthetics. The following technique is employed when there is no damage to the buccal plate; otherwise the use of a barrier membrane, in addition to the bone graft, becomes necessary (GBR). The rationale is that the barrier membrane protects the blood clot, keeps the space for new bone formation, and prevents epithelial and connective tissue cell migration to the area (Gottlow 1994). This enables the bone graft to heal undisturbed in a contained environment.

Bone that is used can be autogenous, allogenic, synthetic, or a xenograft. The only relative contraindication to this technique is active infection at the site of extraction. It is recommended to resolve the infection before grafting the socket. If

a socket preservation in the presence of infection is necessary because of time constraints or other influencing factors, appropriate antibiotic treatment should be started the day before the procedure and be continued for a total of 7 days.

REFERENCES

Antoun, H., Sitbon, J.M., Martinez, H., & Missika, P. (2001) A prospective randomized study comparing two techniques of bone augmentation: Onlay graft alone or associated with a membrane. *Clinical Oral Implants Research* 12, 632–639.

Gottlow, J. (1994) Periodontal regeneration. In: Lang, N.P., & Karring, T., eds. *Proceedings of the First European Workshop on Periodontology.* London: Quintessence, 172–192.

Lekovic, V., Kenney, E.B., Weinlaender, M., Han, T., Klokkevold, P., Nedic, M., & Orsini, M. (1997) A bone regenerative approach to alveolar ridge maintenance following tooth extraction: Report of 10 cases. *Journal of Periodontology* 68, 563–570.

Lekovic, V., Camargo, P.M., KLokkevold, P.R., Weinlaender, M., Kenney, E.B., & Dimitrijevic, B. (1998) Preservation of alveolar bone in extraction sockets using bioabsorbable membranes. *Journal of Periodontology* 69, 1044–1049.

Moore, W.R., Graves, S.E., & Bain, G.I. (2001) Synthetic bone graft substitutes. *Australian & New Zealand Journal of Surgery* 71, 354–355.

Pini-Prato, G.P., Cairo, F., Tinti, C., Cortellini, P., Muzzi, L., & Mancini, E.A. (2004) Prevention of alveolar ridge deformities and reconstruction of lost anatomy: A review of surgical approaches. *International Journal of Periodontics and Restorative Dentistry* 24, 435–445.

Scipioni, A., Bruschi, G.B., & Calesini, G. (1994) The edentulous ridge expansion technique: A five-year study. *International Journal of Periodontics and Restorative Dentistry* 14, 451–459.

Scipioni, A., Bruschi, G.B., Calesini, G., Bruschi, E., & De Martino, C. (1999) Bone regeneration in the edentulous ridge expansion technique: Histologic and ultrastructural study of 20 clinical cases. *International Journal of Periodontics and Restorative Dentistry* 19, 269–277.

Sclar, A.G. (2003) Bio-Col technique for delayed implant placement. In: *Soft Tissue and Esthetic Considerations in Implant Therapy.* Carol Stream, IL: Quintessence, 75–112.

Seibert, J.S. (1983a) Reconstruction of deformed, partially edentulous ridges, using full thickness onlay grafts. Part I. Technique and wound healing. *Compendium of Continuing Education in Dentistry* 4, 437–453.

Seibert, J.S. (1983b) Reconstruction of deformed, partially edentulous ridges, using full thickness onlay grafts. Part II. Prosthetic/periodontal interrelationships. *Compendium of Continuing Education in Dentistry* 4, 549–562.

Summers, R.B. (1994) The osteotome technique. Part 2. The ridge expansion osteotomy (REO) procedure. *Compendium of Continuing Education in Dentistry* 15, 422–426.

Von Arx, T., Cochran, D.L., Herman, J.S., Schenk, R.K., & Buser, D. (2001) Lateral ridge augmentation using different bone fillers and barrier membrane application: A histologic and histomorphometric pilot study in the canine mandible. *Clinical Oral Implants Research* 12, 260–269.

Chapter 13: Exposure of Impacted Maxillary Teeth for Orthodontic Treatment

Serge Dibart

HISTORY

Impactions of the maxillary teeth, canines in particular, can be classified as labial, palatal, and intermediate (Kruger 1984). Precise localization of the crown through intraoral radiographs is important to determine the surgical approach and the flap design.

INDICATION

• Exposure of impacted teeth

ARMAMENTARIUM

This includes the basic kit plus surgical round burrs (carbide or diamond).

TECHNIQUE

After localization of the crown, buccally or palatally, the area is anesthetized. In the case of buccal impaction, it is critical to design the incision to retain as much attached gingiva as possible to avoid a mucogingival defect afterward (Fig. 13.1). A full-thickness flap with vertical releasing incisions is elevated to expose the underlying bony bulge (Fig. 13.2).

At this point, the crown is either only partially visible or not visible. A round burr (no. 4 or no. 6) can be used to expose the crown further. The flap is then apically repositioned and sutured below the exposed crown. An apical sharp dissection may be necessary to enable flap fixation (to the periosteum). After a short healing phase (Fig. 13.3), an orthodontic bracket is secured on the crown for future tooth alignment.

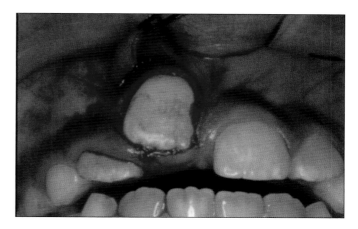

Figure 13.2. The crown is exposed and the flap sutured apically (not shown).

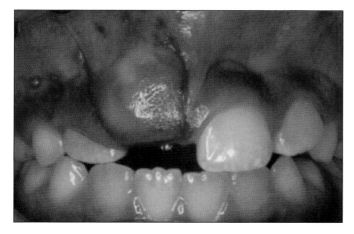

Figure 13.1. A buccal full-thickness flap is elevated to expose the crown of tooth 8.

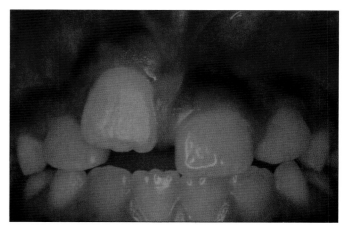

Figure 13.3. Healing after 1 month.

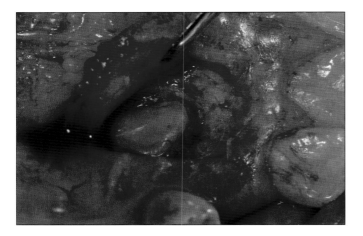

Figure 13.4. A palatal semilunar flap to expose an impacted canine.

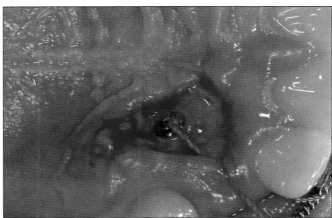

Figure 13.5. The tip of the flap has been trimmed and a bracket placed on the exposed crown.

In case of palatal crown location, a semilunar incision is made on the palate and the crown exposed with or without ostectomy (Fig. 13.4). Since we cannot apically position the flap in the palate, a scissor is used to cut off the tip of the flap and leave the crown exposed. At this point, a bracket is placed on the crown (Fig. 13.5).

REFERENCE

Kruger, G.O. (1984) *Oral and Maxillofacial Surgery*, 6th edition. St. Louis: C.V. Mosby, 91–93.

Chapter 14: Soft Tissue Management Around Dental Implants

Diego Capri

INTRODUCTION

Implant therapy has evolved significantly during the last two decades, from being one of the treatments of choice for edentulous arches to becoming a routine procedure to replace lost dental elements, regardless of the type of edentulism (Adell et al. 1981). With this development, the objective of implant therapy has expanded from the functional restoration of the missing dentition to include the re-creation of the lost hard and soft tissues (Garber & Belser 1995).

Only when a close resemblance with what once existed in nature is achieved does the end result of implant therapy become a success for its ability to provide the proper mas-

ticatory function while disappearing in between the remaining natural teeth.

For an implant restoration to closely mimic the lost dental element, it is undoubtedly important to select the proper shape and color of the prosthetic tooth. Nonetheless, it is imperative to surround the crown with healthy, gingival-like tissue (Figs. 14.1–14.4).

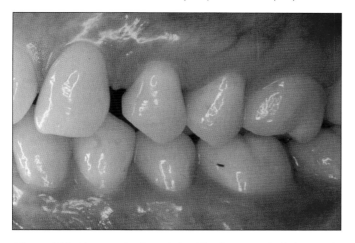

Figure 14.1. Preoperative buccal view. The first premolar is fractured.

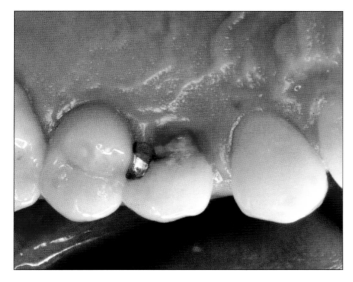

Figure 14.2. Preoperative palatal view. The fracture line extends several millimeters subgingivally.

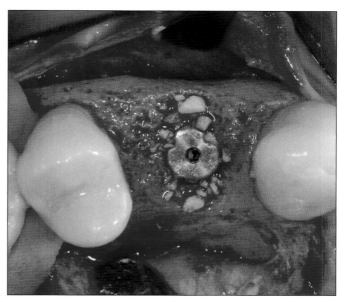

Figure 14.3. At 6 weeks after the extraction, a single implant is placed into the residual socket, and a xenograft is used to fill the voids between the implant and the osseous walls.

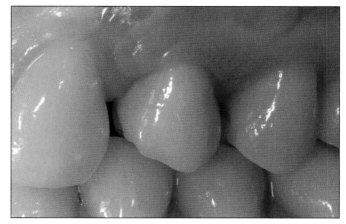

Figure 14.4. The final implant-supported restoration is in place. There is a harmonious integration of the prosthetic crown in between the natural dental elements and the healthy and natural appearance of the peri-implant gingiva.

GINGIVAL TISSUES
AND PERI-IMPLANT MUCOSA

When handling the peri-implant soft tissue, it is important to acknowledge the differences that exist between the peri-implant mucosa and the gingival tissue. The mucosa that encircles the fixture has more collagen and fewer fibroblasts, with a 2:1 ratio, when compared with the periodontal gingival tissue (Berglundh et al. 1991; Abrahamsson et al. 2002).

The collagen fibers of the healthy periodontium are functionally arranged in a complex system (Smukler & Dreyer 1969), which differs from the fiber bundles of the peri-implant mucosa. The system runs mostly parallel to the titanium surface without attaching to it (Berglundh et al. 1991). It has been reported that both the titanium surface's characteristics (Schroeder et al. 1981; Piattelli et al. 1997) and the mobility of the soft tissues (Listgarten et al. 1991) will affect the orientation of the collagen fibers. Nonetheless, even when the fibers are more perpendicularly disposed, there is no real functional insertion.

When compared with the supracrestal vessels of a natural dental element, the supracrestal vascular topography surrounding the fixture is reduced and diversely arranged (Berglundh et al. 1994; Moon et al. 1999). Both the tooth and the implant have a junctional epithelium that is approximately 2 mm long (Berglundh et al. 1991).

Despite the very similar clinical appearance between the peri-implant soft tissue and the gingiva encircling a natural dental element, the histological dissimilarities mentioned earlier bear a great responsibility in the selection of the most appropriate way to manage the peri-implant mucosa.

Encompassing the fixture is tissue, with its lower cellularity and reduced vascularity, that resembles cicatritial tissue and requires special care when surgically challenged. In the basic periodontal wound-healing processes, after flap elevation, one of the most dynamic tissues involved is the periodontal ligament (Goldman & Cohen 1980). The lack of this ligament, with its vessels and cells, must be kept in mind when approaching the peri-implant mucosa.

Although periodontal plastic procedures are used daily to correct peridental sites where mucogingival problems have already occurred, in implant therapy the less forgiving nature of the tissues involved makes it advisable initially to optimize the peri-implant soft tissues to prevent future complications.

The quality and quantity of the peri-implant tissues should be improved either before or at implant placement, during the submerged healing, or at the time of second-stage surgery (Nevins & Mellonig 1998). The outcome of some root-coverage procedures should not be considered as predictable for implants in communication with the oral environment (one-stage implants, uncovered two-stage implants, or implants supporting a prosthesis), as they are around natural teeth (Harris 1994; Sclar 2003).

In an attempt to cover an exposed implant-abutment complex, or to mask the grayishness that transpires through thin peri-implant mucosal tissue, surgical approaches, such as the variously displaced pedicle flaps (coronally, laterally, double papilla, etc.) or free gingival autografts, usually fall short. In such unfortunate clinical scenarios, and provided that the angle of emergence of the implant-abutment-crown complex is not excessively buccal, a coronally advanced flap augmented by a subepithelial connective tissue graft represents the most predictable procedure because of its double blood supply (Langer & Langer 1985; Nelson 1987).

In particularly difficult clinical cases, removing the prosthetic components to resubmerge the fixture can be useful to widen the recipient vascular bed palatally for the subepithelial connective tissue graft. This further increases the predictability of success.

THE NEED FOR KERATINIZED TISSUE

The need for keratinized tissue around the implant is still controversial (Adell et al. 1981; Wennstrom et al. 1994; Warrer et al. 1995). Despite this, the presence of gingival-like tissue has several important advantages. The keratinized gingival tissue provides a tight fibrous collar that surrounds the implant, sealing off the bacteria from the depth of the peri-implant sulcus (Warrer et al. 1995).

The several restorative maneuvers that precede the crown placement are potentially detrimental to tissue health, and the presence of immobile keratinized tissue seems, at least from an immediate clinical perspective, to better withstand the trauma that is caused. Also this allows for easier plaque control for the patient and during periodic maintenance recall visits (Figs. 14.5–14.9).

Peri-implant tissue that resembles the keratinized gingiva on the adjacent natural teeth is important in the aesthetic zone. The free autogenous gingival graft (Sullivan & Atkins 1968) still represents the preferred procedure to predictably increase the keratinized soft tissue that encircles the implant.

The tissue that forms around the transmucosal portion of the implant, though initially considered similar to the dentogingival junction (Berglundh et al. 1991), often limits the predictability of achieving ideal soft tissue profiles. This is particularly true in the interimplant areas, where the presence or absence of the papillae determines the final aesthetic result (Tarnow et al. 2003).

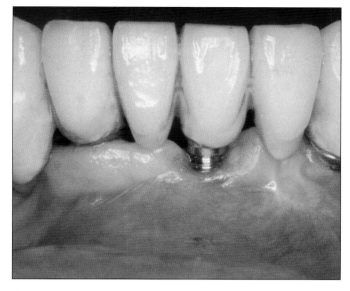

Figure 14.5. Preoperative view. The patient, treated with an implant-supported restoration 12 years ago, now complains about discomfort during daily oral hygiene procedures.

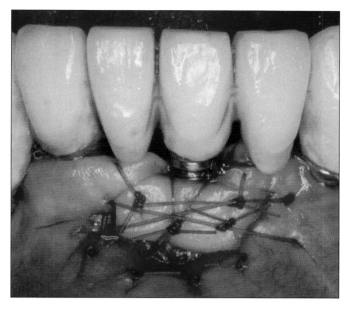

Figure 14.7. A thick, free gingival graft is carefully adapted to the periosteal bed and stabilized with compressive 5-0 gut sutures. No attempt is made to cover the original marginal recession.

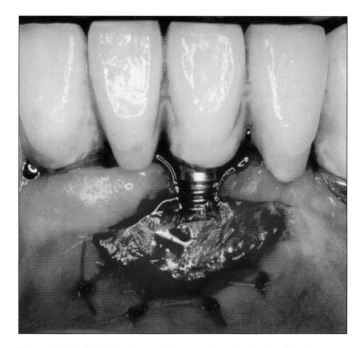

Figure 14.6. A decision is made to use a free gingival graft to increase the amount of keratinized tissue. The main goal is to simplify the home oral hygiene procedures. A periosteal bed has been prepared. There is dehiscence buccal to the otherwise osseointegrated implant.

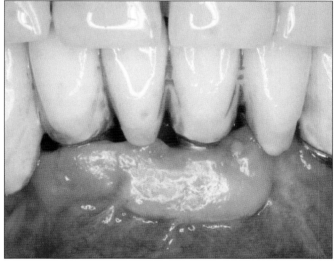

Figure 14.8. Final healing of the area. The patient did not experience any further discomfort during brushing. An unexpected creeping attachment phenomenon of about 2 mm was also obtained.

BIOLOGICAL WIDTH AND GINGIVAL BIOTYPES

This traditionally refers to the sum of two histological peridental entities: the junctional epithelium and the connective tissue attachment (Gargiulo et al. 1961; Vacek et al. 1994). The importance of these two distinct, but related, tissues within the environment of the dentogingival junction has been amply debated in the literature (Maynard & Wilson 1979; Smukler & Chaibi 1997).

The integrity of the dental biological width (average histological value, 2.04 mm) protects, by its biological sealing

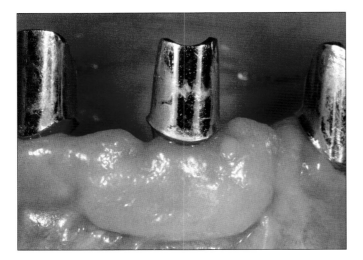

Figure 14.9. After 3 years, during a periodical hygiene recall, stability of the area is evident. The creeping phenomenon progressed for an additional 0.5 mm (compare with Fig. 14.8).

property, the other underlying deep periodontal tissues that are kept separated from the outer oral and sulcular environment (average histological value, 0.69 mm) (Listgarten et al. 1991).

Known for its high histological variability, the biological width together with the gingival sulcus coincide to form the different clinical periodontal biotypes (Weisgold et al. 1997), more recently redefined as periodontal phenotypes (Muller & Eger 2002). The main, and most immediate, clinical expression of the periodontal biotype is related to the degree of scalloping of the gingival tissues. The outline of the gingiva and its scalloping reflect the osseous morphotype of the underlying supporting osseous crest (Vacek et al. 1994).

The dental anatomy, with its convexities and concavities, also affects both the soft and the hard tissues that peak in the tooth surface depressions and fall in areas of surface protuberance (Olsson et al. 1993; Becker et al. 1997; Smukler & Chaibi 1997).

Whereas the gingiva and the osseous crest normally run parallel to each other, and to the tooth cemento-enamel junction buccally and lingually (or palatally) in the interproximal area, the position of the gingival tissues is affected by other variables and may or may not follow the osseous crest profile (Smukler & Chaibi 1997). Factors such as the position of the adjacent dental elements and their anatomy that determine the shape and location of the contact point, together with the interproximal peak of bone, influence papillary form and height (Tarnow et al. 1992).

Under normal circumstances, the height of the soft tissue column, located interproximally, is superior to the height of

the soft tissue column located buccally (Kois 1996). This further magnifies the degree of gingival festooning that tends to flatten out toward the posterior sextants of the mouth. Some authors have speculated on the variation in the extent of the biological width and sulcus depth in the different periodontal biotypes (Muller & Eger 2002).

Despite the academic interest in these observations, it is relevant to remember that, irrespective of the degree of scalloping (periodontal biotype), the biological width of a tooth is invariably located supracrestally. The fibers of the connective tissue attachment, functionally inserted into the cementum as Sharpey's fibers, support the gingival margin and the papilla (Fig. 14.10). In other terms, the papilla, supported by the interproximal peaks of bone, can climb higher as a result of the additional support from the connective tissue attachment to the tooth.

Knowledge of the peculiar histological and anatomical features of the dentogingival junction, which differ from those of the peri-implant mucosa, is fundamental to match the patient's expectations. A clinician must anticipate, before beginning therapy, the potential cosmetic limitations in certain known clinical scenarios.

AESTHETIC PREDICTABILITY

The re-creation of ideal soft tissue profiles (particularly in the papillary areas) around implants is more predictable in areas of single edentulism then in multiple implant sites (Salama et al. 1998; Grunder 2000; Garber et al. 2001; Tarnow et al. 2003) (Figs. 14.11–14.13).

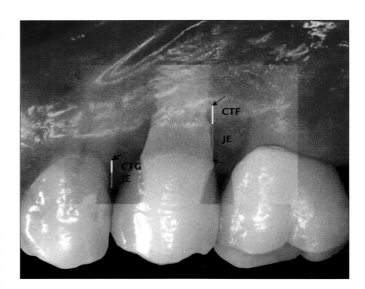

Figure 14.10. The sum of the connective tissue attachment (CTF) and the junctional epithelium (JE) forms the biological width (between the *black arrows*). A biological width around a tooth forms above the crest of bone differently from what we have surrounding an implant where it forms below the level of the bone.

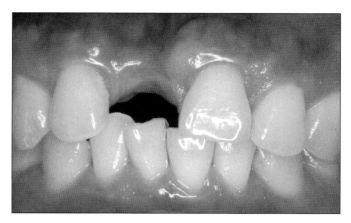

Figure 14.11. Preoperative view. A single implant is planned to replace the missing central incisor. A severe horizontal osseous deficiency was noted at computed tomography, and a chin-graft procedure was selected for the osseous reconstruction prior to implant placement.

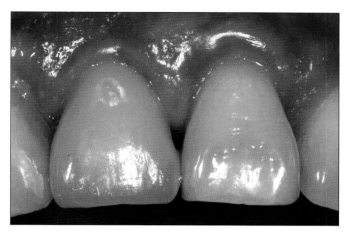

Figure 14.13. Final restoration in place. The patient did not wish to re-create the original diastema with which he was born, and preferred a slight mesiodistal discrepancy between the two centrals. Note the almost ideal gingival scalloping.

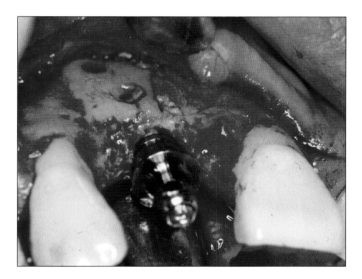

Figure 14.12. The implant is placed 6 months after the osseous augmentation. Note the optimal integration of the osseous autogenous cortical block, easily identifiable in the upper left corner as a result of the two residual bleeding holes remaining after removal of the fixation screws.

Smukler et al. (2003a & b), discussing single implants in the aesthetic zone, stress the difference between the length of interproximal soft tissue on the implant side (4–6.5 mm/implant platform-top of the papilla) and the same distance on the adjacent tooth side (3–4.5 mm/interproximal osseous peak-top of the papilla). It is now widely accepted that, under such clinical circumstances, the interproximal osseous crest on the adjacent natural tooth maintains the height of the papilla (Salama et al. 1998; Grunder 2000; Smukler et al. 2003a & b).

The presence of a thick and flat biotype increases the predictability of a pleasant aesthetic result. Thick tissues are

more resistant to the controlled traumatic injuries caused during dental treatments, and a lower degree of scalloping in the gingiva is more easily replicable at the end of implant therapy. For similar reasons, it is easier to replace a missing tooth in a periodontally treated patient (flat biotype) and obtain soft tissue profiles that are in harmony with the remaining natural dentition (Figs. 14.14–14.16). The possibility of predictably re-creating an ideal gingival outline between two or more contiguous implants has been questioned (Tarnow et al. 2003) (Figs. 14.17–14.22).

Whenever the rehabilitation involves two or more lost teeth, the osseous profile of the edentulous area, matched by the gingival profile, is no longer scalloped but either flat or, even worse, concave. As a result, the precious interproximal osseous septum that normally supports the papilla is no longer available. It is now possible, and advisable, to transform a concave edentulous ridge into a flat one by guided bone regeneration (Simion et al. 1994; Jovanovic & Nevins 1995).

In the best-case scenario, we will start from a flat osseous anatomy into which the implants will be inserted. A proper mesiodistal spacing of the fixtures (at least 3 mm) will grant the maintenance of the interimplant bone height (Salama et al. 1998). This interimplant peak of bone is often more apically located than the one that was present before the loss of the natural dental elements. Additionally, the two contiguous implants do not have Sharpey's fibers functionally inserted into the cementum to support the supracrestal soft tissue (Tarnow et al. 2003).

The biological width around two-stage implants ad modum Brånemark always forms subcrestally (Berglundh & Lindhe 1996). In this process, bone is resorbed (360° around the

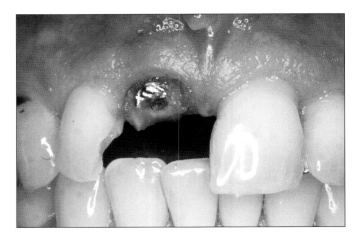

Figure 14.14. Preoperative view. The right central incisor is fractured and scheduled for extraction and immediate implant placement. The crown of the right lateral incisor is fractured as well, and a composite resin restoration will be done. Note the flat and thick biotype and the marginal recession of the gingival tissues.

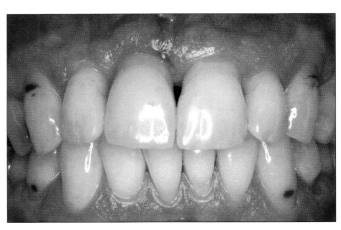

Figure 14.16. Final restoration in place. Despite a slight marginal disharmony between the two centrals, the overall aesthetic result is acceptable because of the generalized gingival recession pattern and the flat biotype of the patient.

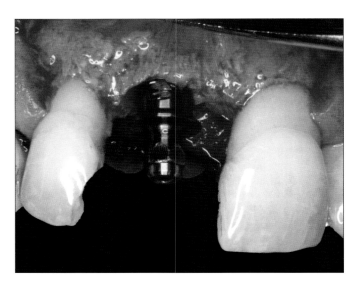

Figure 14.15. Immediate implant placement at the time of extraction.

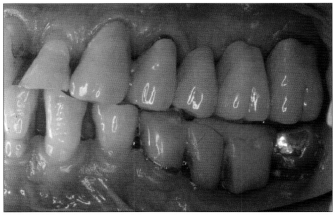

Figure 14.17. Preoperative view of the maxillary and mandibular left sextants. The maxillary first premolar and second molar are hopeless. The second mandibular molar should also be extracted. Multiple implants are planned for both the maxilla and the mandible.

neck of the implant) and replaced by connective tissue fibers. Whether this is the result of the biological width forming (Berglundh & Lindhe 1996) or due to the cupping phenomenon caused by the bacterial contamination of the microgap (Hermann et al. 1997, 2000), the final result does not change. The connective tissue encircles the fixtures subcrestally differently than it does around natural teeth, where the supracrestal connective tissue fibers further support the verticality of the gingival tissue (Tarnow et al. 2003).

When considering that the average height, according to the most recent available data (Tarnow et al. 2003), of the interimplant tissue, measured from the interimplant peak of bone to the tip of the papilla, is 3.4 mm, it is easy to understand the aesthetic limitations encountered when placing two adjacent implants in the cosmetic zone.

ONE-PIECE IMPLANTS VERSUS TWO-PIECE IMPLANTS

Recent investigations of one-piece nonsubmerged implants (ITI implants; Straumann, Basel, Switzerland) have shown different patterns in the way bone heals around the fixture when compared with two piece implants (Hermann et al. 2001). According to the authors, the presence of a microgap in a two-piece implant in the vicinity of the osseous crest

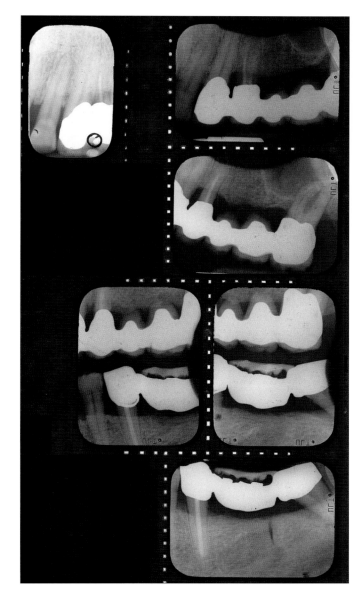

Figure 14.18. Radiographs of the area reveal the extent of the periodontal pathology and the ill-fitting restorations.

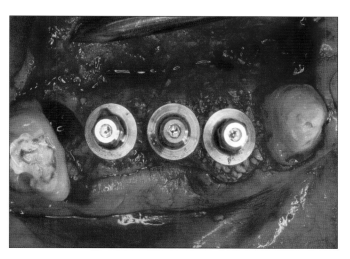

Figure 14.19. Three implants are placed in the maxilla. The first implant, in position of the first premolar, is placed immediately after the removal of the hopeless tooth. The residual socket is grafted with a xenograft. The last implant, in position of the first molar, is placed with a simultaneous sinus elevation by using an osteotome crestal approach. The residual maxillary molar is temporarily retained to support a provisional bridge.

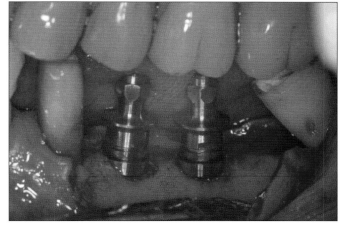

Figure 14.20. Two wide-diameter implants are placed in the mandible while the hopeless mandibular molar is temporarily retained to support the provisional restoration. The patient is asked to close to verify the proper prosthetic position of the fixtures.

would determine an increased resorption of bone when compared with a one-stage one-piece implant (Figs. 14.23–14.26).

In the 1990s, investigations conducted on animals in Sweden demonstrated how multiple disconnections and reconnections of the implant abutment were followed by a more apical relocation of the peri-implant connective tissue band (Abrahamsson et al. 1997). The average biological width measured for a one-piece implant (2.84 mm) would be similar to the width around a natural tooth (2.7 mm + 3 mm = biological width + sulcus depth) and generally smaller than the width measured around a two-piece implant (Ericsson et al. 1996; Hermann et al. 2001). The Brånemark-type of implant would additionally be characterized by a more apical location of the gingival margin when compared with an ITI type of fixture (Hermann et al. 2001).

Despite the evidence presented by the research, which was conducted on a dog model, we must not forget that one-piece, one-stage implants were also included in the investigation conducted by Tarnow et al. (2003) on 136 interimplant papillae measuring an average of 3.4 mm.

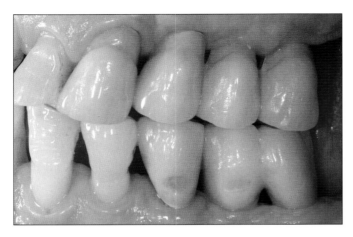

Figure 14.21. Final implant-supported restorations in place. The function of the area was successfully regained with patient satisfaction. Two PFM (porcelain fused to metal) crowns were replaced on the maxillary canine and the mandibular second premolar. There is flatter gingival scalloping and the absence of papillae that are commonly found around multiple adjacent implants.

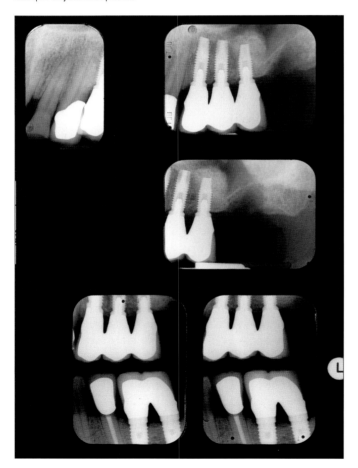

Figure 14.22. Postoperative radiograph. The interimplant peaks of bone were preserved after the 360° peri-implant osseous resorption took place. Despite that, no "real" papillae are clinically present (see Fig. 14.21). The nice radiographic result obtained after simultaneous sinus elevation on the last maxillary implant is clearly visible (compare with Fig. 14.18).

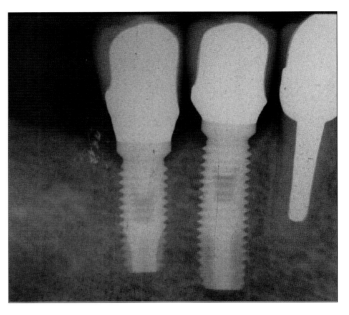

Figure 14.23. Radiograph showing the typical peri-implant osseous resorption pattern around two-piece implants. Usually bone resorbs 360° around the implant platform for a depth of approximately 2 mm.

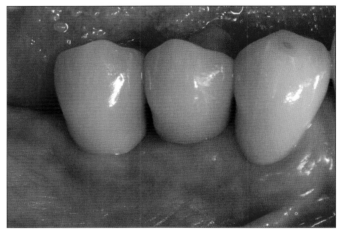

Figure 14.24. Clinical view of the two implants shown in Fig. 14.23.

According to the value reported by Kois (1996), the average papillary height in natural dentition is usually around 4.5 mm, about 1 mm more than measurements between implants. Furthermore, the interimplant peak of bone, despite advancements obtained with osseous regenerative procedures, is commonly found to be more apical than the original interdental osseous crest. This is particularly true in the presence of a scalloped periodontal biotype.

To improve the aesthetic result in the cosmetic zone, the ITI type of fixtures are commonly sunk more apically to obtain transmucosal space that is used to develop an ideal anatomical profile with the prosthetic components that

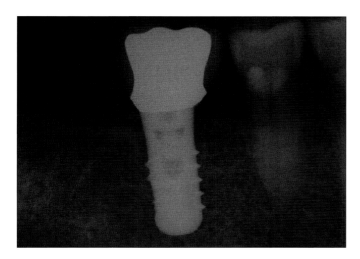

Figure 14.25. Radiograph showing the peri-implant osseous resorption pattern around a one-piece transmucosal implant (compare with Fig. 14.23). Although the resorption pattern is certainly different from that of a two-stage type of implant, a narrower cupping defect is still apparent.

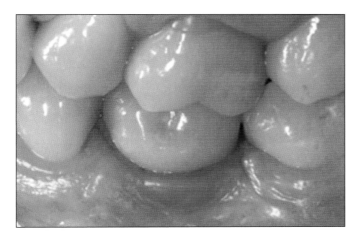

Figure 14.26. Clinical view of the implant shown in Fig. 14.25.

connect to the otherwise unanatomical round platform of the implant. In doing so, the rough-smooth interface of the implant is buried deeper into the bone and, according to the research by Hermann et al. (1997, 2000), this determines a larger circumferential loss of crestal bone. Under these circumstances, the differences, if any, between one-stage or two-stage implants are minimal.

In the attempt to overcome the limitations, new scalloped fixture designs have been proposed (Holt et al. 2002) and recently introduced into the market (Wöhrle 2003). More research is still needed to validate the benefits claimed with the use of the designs.

With the knowledge that crestal bone remodels away, both vertically and horizontally, from the implant-abutment interface (Tarnow et al. 2000), several clinicians have success-

fully managed to minimize the peri-implant osseous cupping by moving the microgap inward. This clinical intuition has been recently defined as the *platform switching* technique and can be easily accomplished (with certain implant types) by downsizing the diameter of the abutment (e.g., 4-mm abutment platform) in relation to the supporting implant diameter (e.g., 5-mm implant platform) (Figs. 14.27–14.29).

In the author's own experience, this still anecdotal, easily performed, clinical trick has been proven to reduce the extent of the peri-implant crestal bone loss significantly, at least from a radiological standpoint (Figs. 14.30 & 14.31).

It is relevant to note how some implant manufacturers have, in the past, designed their fixtures with a coronal bevel that brings the abutment to sit inside the implant platform. Research comparing this latter design (Astra Tech implants; Astra Tech, Waltham, MA, USA) with the more traditional Brånemark fixture produced controversial results regarding differences in the amount of crestal bone resorption (Puchades-Roman et al. 2000; Hermann et al. 2001; Astrand et al. 2004).

Independent from the significance of the compared average values of the vertical osseous loss around the two systems, there was common agreement on the different initial pattern of bone remodeling noted for the beveled platform (Puchades-Roman et al. 2000; Hermann et al. 2001). This observation may lead more implant companies to shape their two-stage implants in such a way that could even out

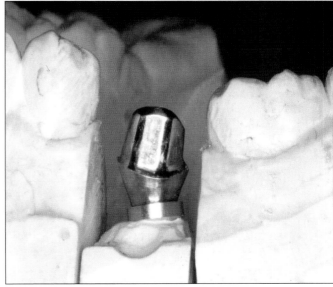

Figure 14.27. According to the platform-switching technique, a 4-mm-diameter abutment is used on a 5-mm-diameter implant platform. In the picture, an anatomical custom abutment has been manufactured.

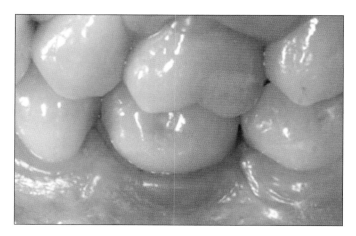

Figure 14.28. Clinical view of the implant shown in Fig. 14.27.

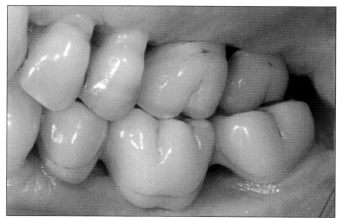

Figure 14.31. Clinical view of the maxillary implants shown in Fig. 14.30.

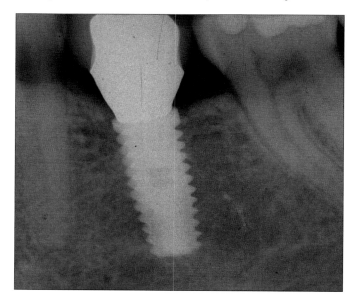

Figure 14.29. Radiograph of the implant depicted in Fig. 14.27. Note how the platform-switching approach seems to abate the amount of peri-implant bone loss.

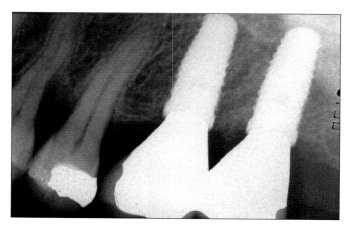

Figure 14.30. Radiograph showing two maxillary implants realized according to the platform-switching concept. No apparent cupping defects are visible.

the discrepancy, in terms of biological width dimensions, with the one-piece transmucosal fixtures (Hermann et al. 2001). It has yet to be determined to what extent this might affect the peri-implant soft tissue profiles and the aesthetic predictability of implants.

UNCOVERING TECHNIQUES

When a submerged approach is selected, a second surgery is performed for several purposes: it enables the implant to be uncovered and verifies the achievement of clinical osseointegration, it enables the healing abutment or the provisional restoration to be connected to the fixture, and it represents the last chance to improve the peri-implant soft tissue. At the second-stage surgery, the site should be carefully evaluated to determine whether the quantity and quality of the soft tissues fulfill the previously planned therapy expectations.

Unfortunately, often deficits in terms of tissue volume, gingival keratinization, or both will be present. Whenever possible, adequate peri-implant keratinized tissue should be obtained by adjacent sites by using pedicle flaps (Moy et al. 1989; Hertel et al. 1994). If the surrounding anatomy does not favor the sculpting of a pedicle flap, the alternative naturally is epithelialized soft tissue grafts (Sullivan & Atkins 1968).

For buccolingual volumetric defects, modifications of the original Abrams's roll technique can be used successfully (Abrams 1980; Scharf & Tarnow 1992; Israelson & Plemons 1993; Barone et al. 1999). The peri-implant soft tissue can also be augmented by grafting connective tissue, either before or at the time of the uncovering (Langer & Calagna 1980; Silverstein et al. 1994; Hurzeler & Weng 1996).

In an attempt to re-create the lost papillary tissues between implants, several techniques have been proposed (Salama et al. 1995; Adriaenssens et al. 1999; Palacci & Ericsson 2001; Tinti & Benfenati 2002; Smukler et al. 2003a). Despite the good clinical intuitions of the authors, the predictability of the different approaches has yet to be scientifically proven.

Other reports address the surgical removal of a nonresorbable membrane during second-stage surgeries (Landi & Sabatucci 2001). The ever-increasing need for guided bone regeneration of implant recipient sites (Grunder et al. 2005) justifies the interest in new uncovering techniques. While the use of new resorbable membranes has mitigated the problems related to barrier removal (Zitzmann et al. 1997; Friedmann et al. 2002), other drawbacks consequential to previous regenerative procedures still deserve some consideration.

The necessity for primary wound closure over a membrane, independent from its biodegradable properties, often results in a coronal displacement of the mucogingival tissues. In many cases, this further reduces the already deficient amount of gingiva that overlies the edentulous ridge and surrounds the adjacent teeth.

New flap designs aimed at minimizing the coronal displacement of the mucogingival junction at the time of membrane placement should be used whenever possible (Tinti & Parma-Benfenati 1995; Nemcovsky et al. 1999, 2000; Triaca et al. 2001). If the anatomy of the treated area does not permit the use of such techniques, the second-stage surgery should be aimed at compensating for the lost mucogingival relationship (Rosenquist 1997). This means using well-known periodontal plastic procedures (repositioned pedicle flaps, free gingival grafts, connective tissue grafts, and the like) to regain the proper lost anatomical landmarks (Figs. 14.32–14.43).

TISSUE-PUNCH UNCOVERING TECHNIQUE

This approach finds its origin in the original description of the second-stage surgery by Dr. P.-I. Brånemark (Garber & Belser 1995). The technique was originally devised for implant-supported restorations of fully edentulous patients and did not consider the final aesthetic outcome of the peri-implant soft tissues (Figs. 14.44 & 14.45).

To quote Rosenquist (1997) regarding the aesthetics of the gingival tissues that abut an implant, "Four factors are important: 1) the width and position of the attached gingiva; 2) the buccal volume of the alveolar process; 3) the level and configuration of the gingival margin; and 4) the size and shape of the papillae."

This approach, which presents the unique advantage of exposing only the head of the implant, thus minimizing the surgical trauma, is indicated only in ideal circumstances

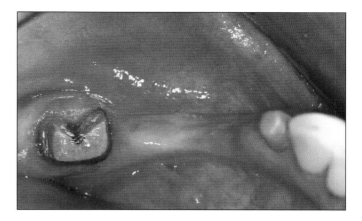

Figure 14.32. Preoperative view of the area planned for an implant-supported restoration. There is a lack of proper bone width in the edentulous area.

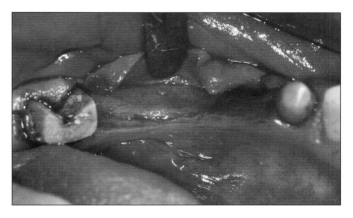

Figure 14.33. After reflection of a full-thickness flap, the deficient buccolingual width of the edentulous ridge is obvious.

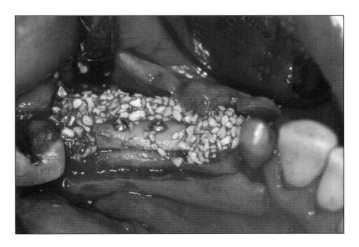

Figure 14.34. A block graft taken from the mandibular ramus, immediately posterior to the area, is secured in place with two fixation screws. Additional particulate xenograft is used to fill the voids and increase the volume of the graft.

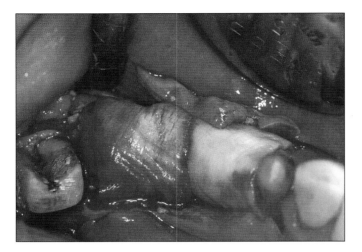

Figure 14.35. A resorbable collagen membrane is used on top of the graft.

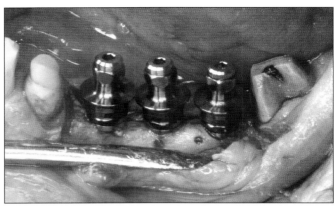

Figure 14.38. Three standard-diameter implants are placed.

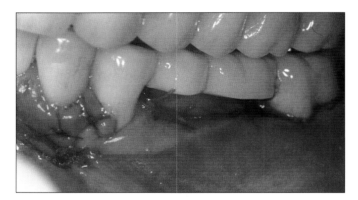

Figure 14.36. After periosteal releasing incisions, primary closure of the wound is achieved. In this maneuver, the mucogingival line is displaced coronally. Note how the provisional restoration has been adjusted to compensate for swelling in the area.

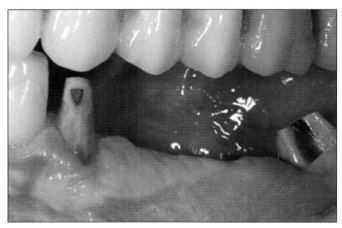

Figure 14.39. The day of the uncovering. The coronal displacement of the mucogingival line, in the edentulous space immediately mesial to the residual second molar, is still noticeable.

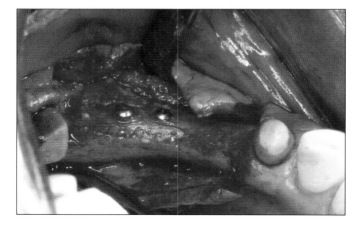

Figure 14.37. After 6 months of healing, the area is reopened. There is excellent graft integration and successful osseous regeneration.

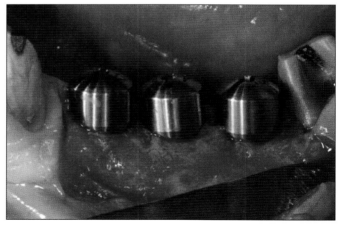

Figure 14.40. A partial thickness flap is reflected, and the temporary healing abutments are placed.

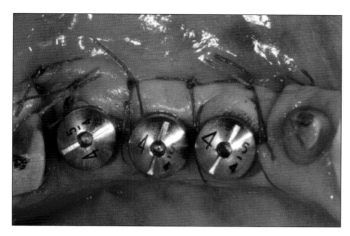

Figure 14.41. The flap is buccally and apically repositioned with 5-0 vicryl, external mattress sutures. Single interrupted sutures are used to close the two vertical releasing incisions. The mucogingival line has been newly moved toward its original, more apical, position.

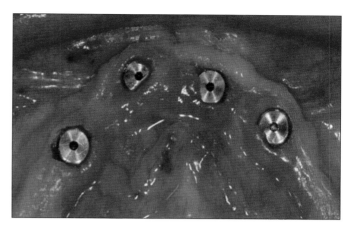

Figure 14.44. Four implants were previously placed in a fully edentulous mandible to support a mandibular overdenture. The uncovering is performed with a no. 15C blade to make circular incisions around the implant platforms.

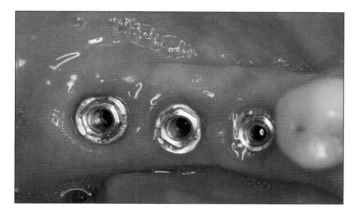

Figure 14.42. After healing of the area, the width of the ridge appears significantly increased as a result of the osseous augmentation (compare with Fig. 14.32). The uncovering technique provided the fixtures with an adequate amount of keratinized mucosa surrounding them. By 4 weeks after the second-stage surgery, there is good healing of the area.

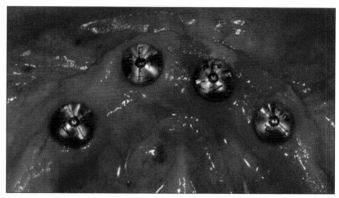

Figure 14.45. The healing abutments are placed, and a gingivoplasty is done, with a diamond round burr, to better harmonize the gingival contours. In such a case, aesthetics is obviously not a priority.

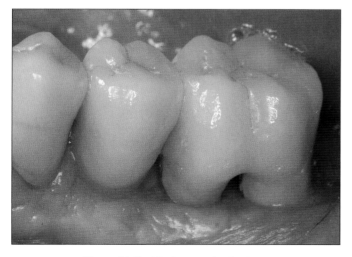

Figure 14.43. Final restoration in place.

(Figs. 14.46 & 14.47). In any other case, the use of a tissue-punch approach would further reduce an already deficient width of keratinized gingiva and make it impossible to correct soft tissue discrepancies.

Another drawback is that, with the tissue punch, the implant/bone interface is not visible and, due to the bleeding, evaluating the proper seating of the abutment can be more difficult. Peri-implant osseous resorptions that developed during the healing after first-stage surgery can go undiagnosed, and a radiograph must be taken to verify that the abutment is seated correctly.

This procedure, which does not require any suturing, causes minimal postoperative discomfort for patients, who may start brushing the area right away. It can easily be accomplished with a dedicated punch-blade.

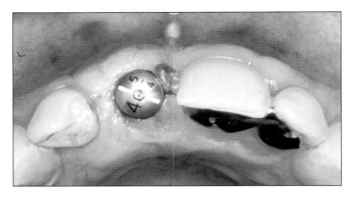

Figure 14.46. In this maxillary anterior case, aesthetics is an important component in obtaining a final successful result. The ideal quality and quantity of the peri-implant mucosal tissues allowed the selection of a tissue-punch technique.

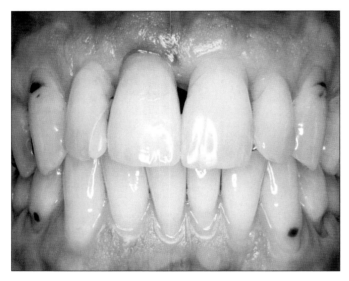

Figure 14.47. The temporary crown is positioned as soon as possible after the tissue punch. In the picture, the temporary is placed 2–3 weeks after the uncovering. There is gingival redness, probably as a result of accidental trauma, buccal to the implant crown. Compare with the finished, final result depicted in Fig. 14.16.

APICALLY POSITIONED FLAP

The transposition of periodontal surgical techniques to implant uncovering procedures seems a natural evolution in the emerging field of implant therapy (Moy et al. 1989). As previously mentioned, the presence of keratinized tissue surrounding implants, although not fundamental for the survival of the fixture, is supported by biological (Nevins & Mellonig 1998), functional (Alpert 1994), and aesthetic factors (Saadoun & LeGall 1992).

The significance of the depth of the peri-implant sulcus has been the object of many investigations. From the initial clinical research that minimized the clinical significance of peri-implant probing depth (Apse et al. 1991), we advanced to awareness of its importance in preventing and avoiding biological complications (Lang et al. 2000). It has been shown that a shallow peri-implant sulcus corresponds with microbial flora distinctive of soft tissue health and vice versa (Dharmar et al. 1994).

Based on the aforementioned considerations, obtaining a firm band of keratinized tissue surrounding a fixture that has a reduced depth of the peri-implant sulcus is today regarded as ideal. The surgical apical repositioning of the gingiva at the time of second-stage surgery is aimed at creating this ideal scenario.

The biological price of this more invasive approach is counterbalanced by several advantages: it provides better access to the implant site, enabling confirmation of the correct seating of the abutment; the soft tissues can be properly thinned, reducing future probing depth; and the keratinized tissue can be preserved or even augmented.

The technique is relatively easy, although more demanding than the punch approach. The author favors the use of a no. 15C blade to sculpt a rectangular, or vaguely trapezoidal, partial thickness flap. This exposes the implant platform onto which the abutment is then placed and is sutured apically to the implant's head (Figs. 14.48–14.50).

The use of a partial thickness flap minimizes the insult to the underlying, often thin, peri-implant osseous anatomy (Staffileno et al. 1966) and enables easier control of flap repositioning as a result of periosteal suturing.

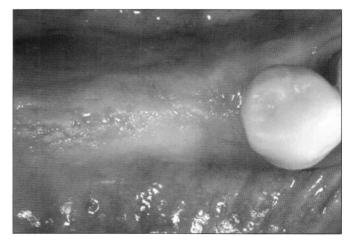

Figure 14.48. Preoperative view. Two implants are buried under the tissue. Note the position of the mucogingival line; an apical repositioning of the keratinized mucosa is needed to idealize the quality of the tissue surrounding the implants.

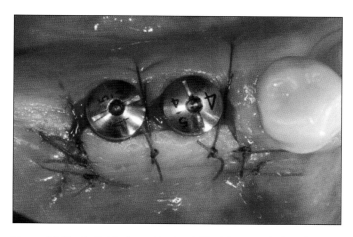

Figure 14.49. A slightly lingual horizontal incision was designed, sparing the papilla distal to the premolar. Two beveled vertical releasing incisions have been placed, mesial and distal to the first incision, and a partial thickness flap has been raised. After positioning the two healing abutments, the flap is sutured apical to its original location.

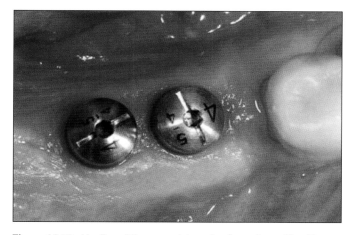

Figure 14.50. Healing of the area at 4 weeks. A good quantity of keratinized mucosa surrounds the fixtures.

For single implants, the two vertical releasing incisions are usually kept slightly divergent toward the buccal vestibule to provide for better blood supply to the narrower coronal portion of the partial thickness flap (Mormann & Ciancio 1977). The vertical incisions are beveled to improve the healing, reduce the scarring, and ease the adaptation of the flap onto its underlying vascular bed (Saadoun & LeGall 1992).

Avoid the inclusion of the papillae in the flap whenever the mesiodistal space of the edentulous area is larger than 6 mm (Saadoun 1997). Although including the papillary areas in the flap would not impair the final formation of nice papillae, if the osseous septum is properly located (Smukler et al. 2003a) their exclusion from the flap design

enables immediately mature interproximal tissue to be readily molded by the provisional restoration (Tarnow et al. 2003).

When the mesiodistal space is too constricted (6 mm), it becomes difficult to design a flap properly that spares the papillae, and the coronal portion of the flap will become extremely narrow with a high risk of necrosis. When the technique is used to uncover multiple implants, the two vertical releasing incisions are kept parallel to each other and beveled, as already described. This simplifies the apical sliding of this more rectangular flap in comparison with the previously described trapezoidal flap.

For the second-stage surgery of two or more implants, the broader extent of the flap crossed by numerous blood vessels, providing the proper nutrition, is such that its base need not be widened to enrich the blood flow. These multiple implant flaps are designed so that the papillae of the adjacent teeth can usually be spared.

One of the main goals in using an apically positioned flap is to preserve or increase the amount of keratinized tissue buccal to the fixture(s). The more the crestal incision is positioned toward the palatal/lingual, the more keratinized tissue is moved apically and buccally to the implant(s). In the mandible, moving the incision lingually is often more limited because the keratinization of the edentulous areas is usually reduced. There is no real advantage in completely depriving the lingual side of keratinized gingiva to slide it buccally.

In the maxilla, a greater source of keratinized tissue is in the palatal vault. When the crestal incision is then pushed toward the palatal side, more bone may be left exposed in this area. Techniques have been described by Tinti & Benfenati (2002) and by Nemcovsky et al. (1999) to obtain tissue from the remaining palatal mucosa to cover the osseous exposure. One often finds that the palate is thick enough to start splitting the flap at the level of the crestopalatal incision so as to leave a protective periosteal layer bound to the palatal bone and interproximally to the implants (Figs. 14.51–14.53).

When the crestal incision falls within the confines of the implant head(s), the remaining portion of the platform is easily exposed by a semilunar incision. When designing the crestopalatal split-thickness flap, overextend it in the mesiodistal direction (see Fig. 14.53). The wider transverse diameter of the buccal convexity of the maxillary alveolar process, compared with the smaller transverse diameter of the palatal concavity of the alveolar process, tends to increase the mesiodistal width of the vestibular recipient bed onto which the palatal mucosa is apically and buccally moved. Not to consider this will often result in a coronal pedicle narrower than its recipient bed and

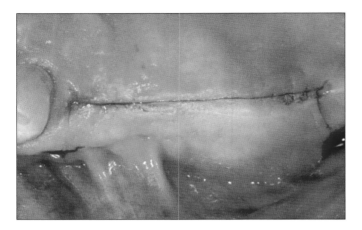

Figure 14.51. A crestopalatal incision is placed to uncover three maxillary implants.

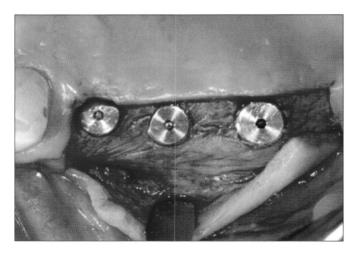

Figure 14.52. The splitting of the flap starts immediately at the level of the crestopalatal incision, leaving the inter-implant periosteum in place. A slight semilunar incision is done to expose the mesial implant further.

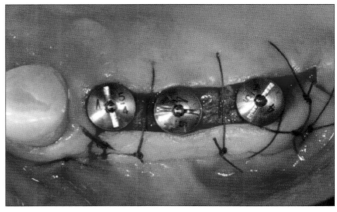

Figure 14.53. The flap is apically positioned with periosteal single interrupted sutures. A crossed-sling suture is used to obtain a tighter adaptation of the keratinized tissue buccally to the distal implant. A standard 4.1-mm-diameter temporary healing abutment is placed on the distal fixture that instead has a 5 mm diameter according to the platform-switching concept.

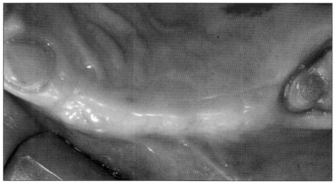

Figure 14.54. Preoperative view of an area where four implants were previously placed.

thus not properly covering the mesiodistal extension of the implant(s). This problem becomes even more significant if the two vertical releasing incisions are kept divergent toward the vestibule rather than parallel to each other.

Once the healing abutments have been seated and checked for proper positioning on the implant platforms, suturing begins. Flap stabilization in its new apical and buccal position is greatly enhanced by the presence of the buccal periosteal layer, onto which the sutures are anchored. Usually single interrupted sutures or external vertical or horizontal mattresses are used to close the wound.

This approach can be further modified using the palatal mucosa as a source of little pedicles that are interproximally rotated similarly to what was originally described by

Pallacci (Scharf & Tarnow 1992). This often accelerates the healing of the interproximal areas molded by the anatomical emergence profiles of the abutment-crown complexes (Figs. 14.54–14.57).

Sometimes, in the posterior maxilla in conjunction with the apically repositioned flap, the thickness of the residual tissue palatal to the implants requires further thinning accomplished in a fashion similar to periodontal pocket-elimination surgery. This is in combination with the goal of reducing the final palatal peri-implant probing depth.

BUCCALLY POSITIONED ENVELOPE FLAP

This approach, designed by Hyman Smukler and colleagues (2003a & b), represents, in its simplicity of execu-

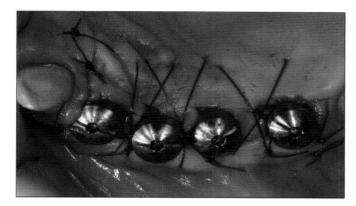

Figure 14.55. Little triangular pedicles obtained from the mucosa palatal to the three last distal implants are interproximally rotated and stabilized in position by crossed horizontal external mattress sutures.

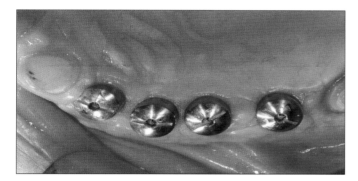

Figure 14.56. Postoperative healing of the area 4 weeks after the uncovering. There is good maturation of the inter-implant tissues.

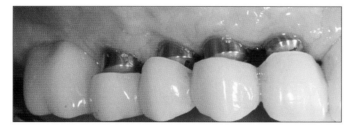

Figure 14.57. Buccal view of postoperative healing of the area 4 weeks after the uncovering. There is good maturation of the interproximal areas and an adequate scalloped soft tissue profile. The provisional restoration was modified to make room for the temporary healing abutments.

tion, a brilliant attempt to idealize the peri-implant soft tissue profiles surgically (Figs. 14.58–14.64). It is best indicated for single implants in the aesthetic zone, even though it can be used for multiple implants.

Use a no. 15C blade to draw a straight incision from the palatal line angle of the mesial dental element to the palatal

line angle of the distal one. A full-thickness envelope flap is raised buccally after intrasulcular incisions are placed on each adjacent tooth.

Vertical releasing incisions should not be used. The buccal portion of the cover screw is now visible, and a semilunar palatal incision is placed to fully expose the implant platform and enable proper seating of the healing abutment, or better, of the provisional restoration, when available.

The flap is held standing in its buccal position by the healing abutment or provisional crown. Two horizontal internal mattress sutures are then placed at the base of each papilla to stabilize the flap and avoid compression on the papillary areas. Design the buccal gingival scallop with a fresh no. 15C blade and draw the proposed buccal gingival margin at a more coronal level than the ones on the adjacent teeth. This is done to obtain an excess of buccal tissue, which will be fine-tuned by the anatomically designed temporary restoration. Keep in mind that a certain degree of apical recession is normally expected (Grunder 2000).

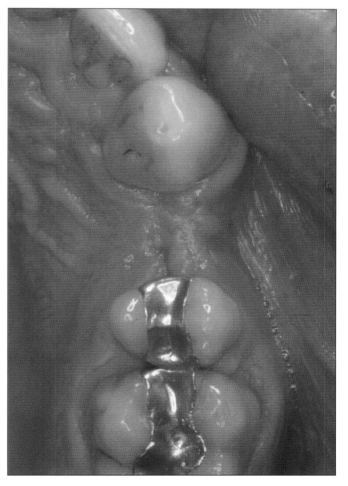

Figure 14.58. Preoperative view of the area to be uncovered. Together with a buccally positioned envelope flap, a connective tissue graft is planned to plump up the buccal ridge.

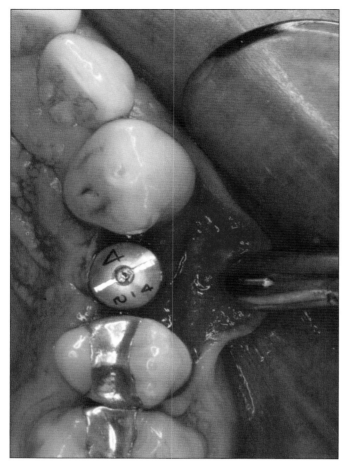

Figure 14.59. A straight incision is designed from the palatal line angle of the canine to the palatal line angle of the premolar. No vertical releases are placed. After the reflection of a full-thickness buccal flap, the temporary abutment is seated.

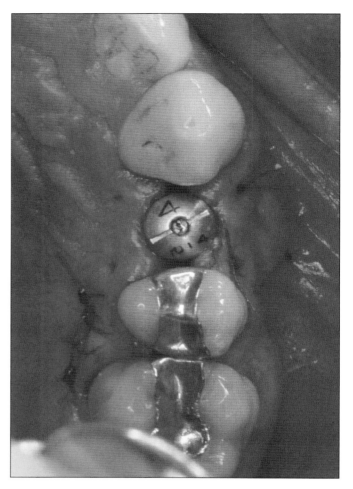

Figure 14.60. After removing the excessive palatal mucosa with a semilunar incision for better tissue adaptation around the temporary abutment, a connective tissue graft is taken from the adjacent palate. The graft is tucked under the buccal envelope flap, and internal horizontal mattress sutures are placed in the interproximal areas.

A two-stage surgical approach similar to the one just described has been proposed by Tinti & Benfenati (2002) to obtain papillae between multiple implants in the aesthetic zone. For these techniques to succeed, it is important to evaluate preoperatively the amount of buccal keratinized tissue available.

If the area has a lack of buccal gingival tissue, there is a risk of further reducing the tissue. Under this circumstance, either select a different approach (i.e., apically positioned flap) or augment the keratinized tissue (i.e., free gingival graft) before proceeding with the buccally positioned envelope flap.

CONNECTIVE TISSUE GRAFT

Use a subepithelial connective tissue graft (Langer & Calagna 1980) during stage-one surgery to build up the ridge volume buccolingually and/or apicocoronally. At uncovering, the placement of the healing screw or of the temporary crown precludes the use of a connective tissue graft to plump up the area coronally.

During second-stage surgery, however, such a graft can be used to augment the buccolingual volume of the ridge, creating the illusion of a root prominence, increasing the gingival thickness, and generally improving the final aesthetic result (Figs. 14.65–14.70). For certain edentulous spaces with major contour deficiencies, soft tissue grafting can be repeated several times (stage-one surgery, stage-two surgery, and between the two stages) to achieve the desired result. Multiple grafts are possible, within the same surgical procedure, from several donor sites and strategically positioned where most needed.

The recipient site is prepared in a similar fashion as traditional periodontal root-coverage procedures. It is always preferred to design the incision by splitting the periosteum

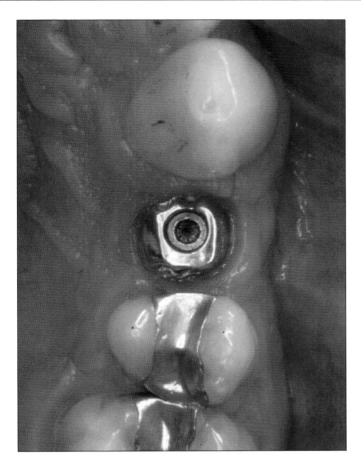

Figure 14.61. Postoperative occlusal view of the area. The buccal concavity has disappeared (compare with Fig. 14.58).

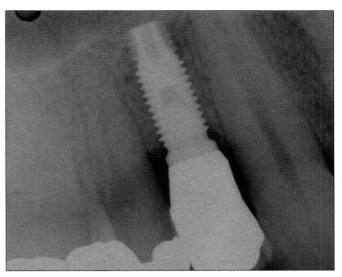

Figure 14.63. The x-ray of the implant reveals a lower interproximal height of bone to support the distal papilla.

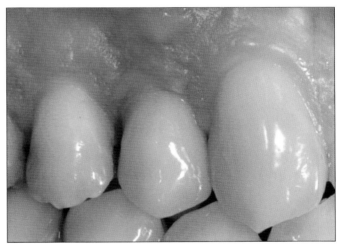

Figure 14.64. Follow-up of the case at 3 years.

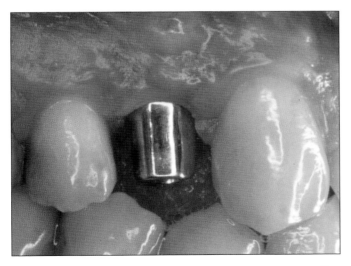

Figure 14.62. Postoperative buccal view of the area. The distal papilla may not be ideal because of the lack of adequate interproximal osseous support in the area (see Fig. 14.63).

to maintain the osseous periosteal coverage as an additional source of nourishment for the subepithelial connective tissue graft. However, when grafting the area during implant placement (stage-one surgery), the graft can be placed between the osseous surface, denuded by a full-thickness flap, and the flap itself.

During uncovering procedures, a no. 15C blade is used to draw a straight, or slightly scalloped, crestal incision that continues in the interproximal and buccal sulci of each adjacent tooth. A partial thickness buccal flap is obtained by severing the periosteum well beyond the mucogingival line while not perforating the vestibular tissue. Vertical releasing incisions are not necessary.

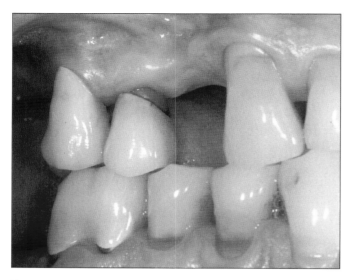

Figure 14.65. A single implant was previously placed to replace the missing first premolar. There is a slight buccal concavity in the edentulous area.

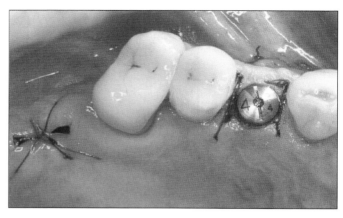

Figure 14.67. The implant was uncovered after reflecting an envelope flap buccally and with a semilunar palatal incision. The connective tissue was taken from the palate distal to the molar and secured under the buccal flap. Single interrupted sutures close the papillary areas while a crossed horizontal mattress is used to close the donor site.

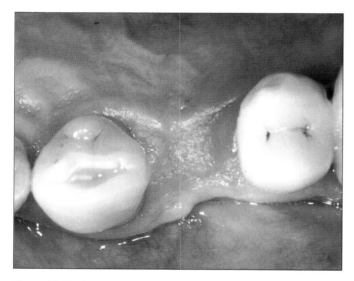

Figure 14.66. An occlusal view of the edentulous space better shows the buccal concavity. During uncovering, a connective tissue graft will be positioned to fill the void.

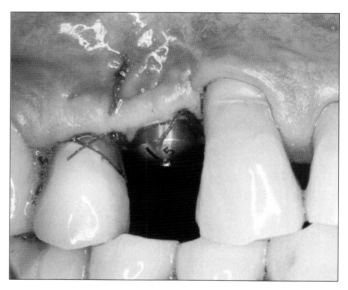

Figure 14.68. The connective tissue graft is better stabilized under the buccal envelope flap with a suture that is visible in the buccal mucosa. The buccal concavity has been filled (see Fig. 14.65).

Design a semilunar incision to uncover the palatal portion of the cover screw from the remaining covering tissue to enable the seating of the prosthetic components. The palatal mucosa, surrounding the implant platform, is usually not reflected unless its thickness exceeds 4 mm. When this is the case, reflecting the palatal tissue thins it while simultaneously collecting the connective tissue graft from the inner portion of the palatal flap.

The graft is secured buccally to the periosteum by using single interrupted resorbable 5-0 gut, or vicryl, sutures.

The collected connective tissue can also be secured by suturing it with an internal horizontal mattress suture to the inner aspect of the vestibular flap, always keeping the knot on the outer buccal surface of the flap.

When the thinning of the mucosa, immediately palatal to the implant, is not needed, the donor site is prepared as originally described by Bruno in 1994. Always in the palate, 2 to 3 mm below the gingival margin of the adjacent posterior teeth, a straight incision is first placed at a 90° angle to the teeth and down to the bone.

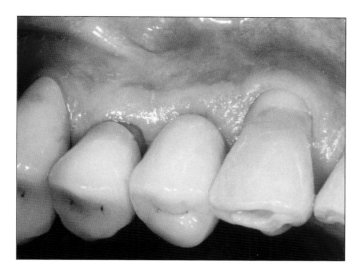

Figure 14.69. The final crown is in place. The soft tissue anatomy has been idealized. No soft tissue concavity can be seen buccally to the implant.

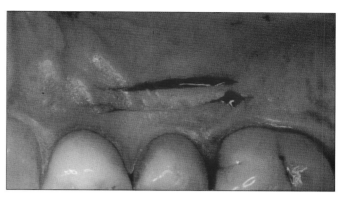

Figure 14.71. Two parallel incisions are drawn in the palate: the coronal one at a 90° angle to the teeth and the apical one (usually the bleeding one) almost parallel to the teeth. The area between the mesial portion of the first molar and the distal of the canine is the safest zone from which to collect a graft without encountering the palatine artery.

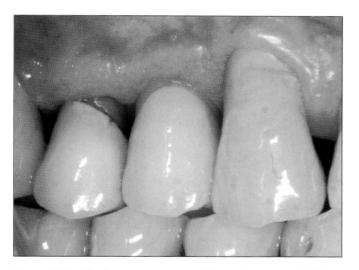

Figure 14.70. The final crown is in place. The patient, pleased with the result, refused to have the crown on the second bicuspid replaced to improve the aesthetics of the area further.

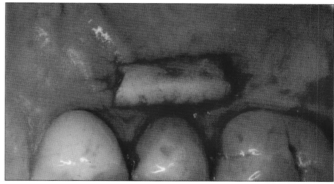

Figure 14.72. After placing two lateral incisions, one mesial and one distal to the first two parallel ones, a wedge of connective tissue can be detached from the palate.

A second, more apical incision, parallel to the first one, is then drawn, this time keeping the blade parallel to the long axis of the teeth (Fig. 14.71). The distance between the two incision lines determines the graft thickness; the closer the space between the parallel lines, the thinner is the graft and vice versa.

Once the palatal incisions are placed, a periosteal elevator is introduced into the most coronal incision to dissect a full-thickness wedge of connective tissue. To detach the graft fully, place two additional lateral incisions, entering with the no. 15C blade between the two parallel lines, first mesially and then distally to the wedge of tissue (Fig. 14.72). To facilitate the execution of these last two lateral incisions, it is useful to overextend the two initial parallel incision lines slightly for more space to enter and maneuver the blade.

After removal of the soft tissue from the donor site, the remaining epithelial layer is dissected from the graft while the palatal wound is closed by using either a suspended horizontal crossed suture or a crossed horizontal external mattress suture. The connective tissue graft may also be obtained in the retromolar tuberosity area in a fashion similar to designing a distal wedge during periodontal surgery. Once the graft is sutured into place, the previously raised buccal envelope flap is adapted on top of it by horizontal or vertical internal mattress suturing.

The connective tissue graft approach represents an extremely versatile procedure. It is often executed in association with an apically positioned flap or together with a buccally positioned envelope flap.

MODIFIED ROLL TECHNIQUE

Use this relatively easy procedure in the maxilla to obtain a localized increase in the soft tissue volume buccal to the implant(s) (Abrams 1980; Scharf & Tarnow 1992; Israelson & Plemons 1993; Barone et al. 1999) (Figs. 14.73–14.78). The first straight crestal incision is kept palatal to the head of the implant(s), orienting the scalpel so as to obtain a long external bevel that extends down to the bone. Two vertical releasing incisions are drawn starting from the palatine bevel, sparing the interproximal papillae, and extending past the mucogingival line.

A small periosteal elevator, entering from the vertical releasing incisions, is then used to carefully buccally reflect a full-thickness flap together with its palatine tail. This usually requires some delicacy to avoid tearing and damaging the palatine tail connected to the buccal flap. The epithelial layer of the flap, palatal to the head of the fixture(s), is then sliced off with a sharp no. 15C blade. The palatal portion of this long-tailed flap is then rolled and tucked under the buccal flap.

At times, the flap thickness is such that it becomes difficult to tuck the most palatal portion of it under the buccal flap. To ease this maneuver, either slightly thin the tissue, decreasing the amount of volumetric increase that will be eventually obtained in the area, or place a horizontal partial thickness releasing incision exactly where the tissue should bend under the vestibular flap.

Use a horizontal internal mattress suture to maintain the position of the rolled tissue. After seating of the healing abutment(s), use additional single interrupted sutures to

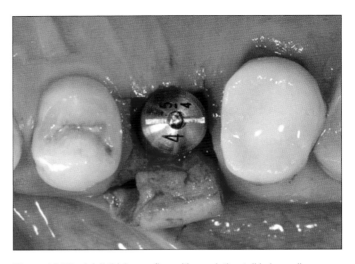

Figure 14.74. A full-thickness flap with a palatine tail is buccally reflected.

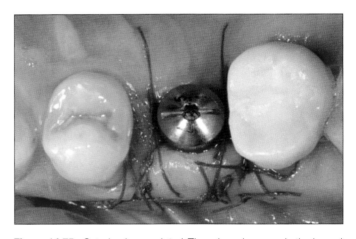

Figure 14.75. Suturing is completed. There is an increase in the buccal volume of tissue (compare with Fig. 14.73).

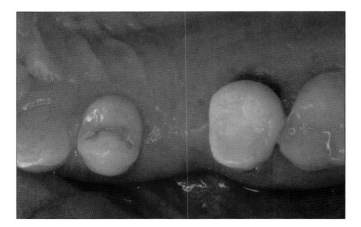

Figure 14.73. Preoperative view of the area. The mesiobuccal root of the first maxillary molar, now wearing a provisional crown, was previously resected for periodontal reasons. An implant was placed in the edentulous space of the missing second premolar. Note the buccal concavity.

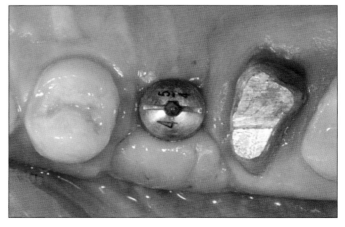

Figure 14.76. Early healing in the area.

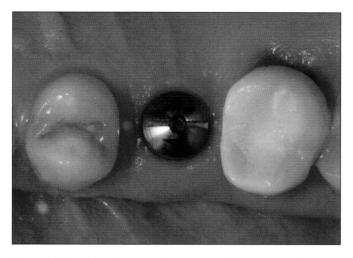

Figure 14.77. Mature healing in the area. A soft tissue convexity visible buccal to the implant simulates a root prominence.

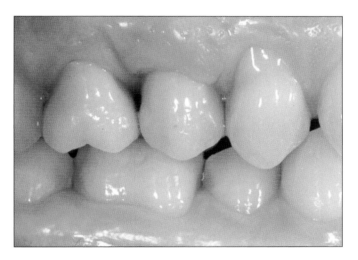

Figure 14.78. Completed case with final restorations on the root resected maxillary molar and on the implant replacing the second premolar.

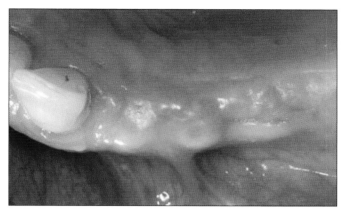

Figure 14.79. Preoperative view of the area to be uncovered. Three implants are buried under the tissue. The thickness of the edentulous ridge is reduced.

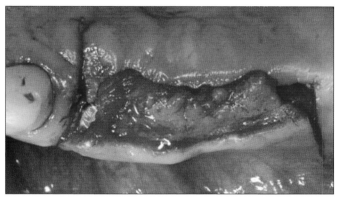

Figure 14.80. A modified roll technique is selected to uncover the three implants. To simplify the procedure, a vertical palatal release is placed, and the flap with its palatine connective tissue tail is buccally reflected.

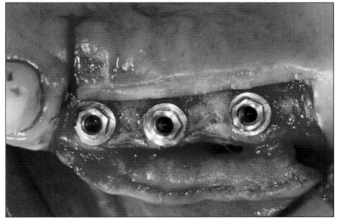

Figure 14.81. The tail is tucked under the buccal flap to increase the buccal thickness of tissue while simultaneously reducing the thickness of the palatal tissue. With this technique, the volume of tissue is increased where it is most needed for aesthetics, and the peri-implant palatal probings are reduced.

close the vertical incisions. Place external vertical mattress sutures to adapt the rolled flap properly to the osseous ridge (Figs. 14.79–14.83).

FREE GINGIVAL GRAFT

This approach continues to represent the gold standard in augmenting the quantity of keratinized tissue surrounding a fixture (Alpert 1994) (Figs. 14.84–14.88). The surgical technique does not substantially differentiate from what is done around natural teeth (Sullivan & Atkins 1968).

Create a recipient periosteal bed with a no. 15C blade around the implant previously exposed with a punch-blade approach. In preparing the recipient bed, it is important to

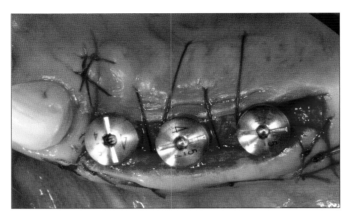

Figure 14.82. While single interrupted sutures close the vertical releasing incisions, combined internal (buccally) and external (palatally) mattress sutures close the interimplant areas. As a result, the buccal flap is held up against the healing abutments while compressing the connective tissue tail, and the thinned palatal flap is compressed down against the palatal bone. This kind of suturing will produce a ramp in the soft tissue from the buccal side toward the palate.

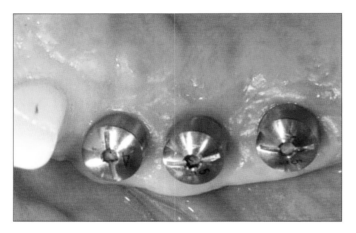

Figure 14.83. Final healing of the area. Note the increase in the volume of soft tissue buccal to the implants and the thin tissue palatal to the fixtures (compare with Fig. 14.79).

completely dissect all of the elastic and muscular fibers. Failure to do so will result in an island of still movable, albeit keratinized, tissue. To increase the firmness of the adherence of the free gingival graft to the underlying recipient bed, the periosteum is additionally scored down to the bone with the scalpel to expose little strips of osseous tissue in the recipient area (Dordick et al. 1976).

Once the recipient area is prepared, the donor site is chosen. Potential donor zones are the palatal mucosa between the first molar and the first premolar, other edentulous ridges, the tuberosity area, and, if there is enough keratinized tissue, the posterior maxillary buccal ridge. The latter area usually offers the best blending tissue for good aesthetic results.

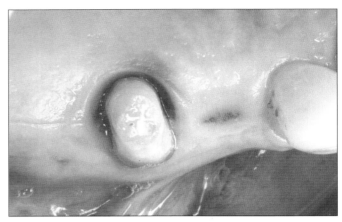

Figure 14.84. Preoperative view. Two implants to be uncovered: one between the canine and the prepared second premolar (planned for extraction) and one distal to the premolar.

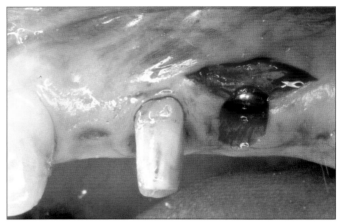

Figure 14.85. A free gingival graft is planned buccal to the distal implant. A periosteal bed is prepared, and the remaining palatal portion of the platform is exposed with a semilunar incision.

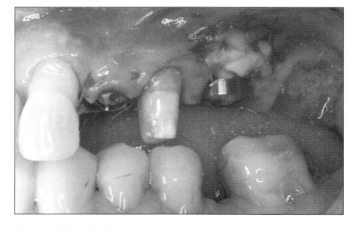

Figure 14.86. The free gingival graft is collected in the posterior maxillary buccal ridge and sutured in its recipient bed buccal to the distal implant. A buccally positioned envelope flap is used to uncover the mesial implant. Resorbable 5-0 gut sutures are used.

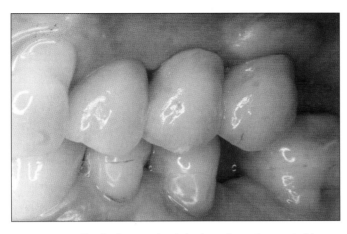

Figure 14.87. The final restoration is in place. A good amount of keratinized mucosa is vestibular to the distal implant. The second premolar was extracted and a three-unit fixed prosthesis supported by the two implants is in place.

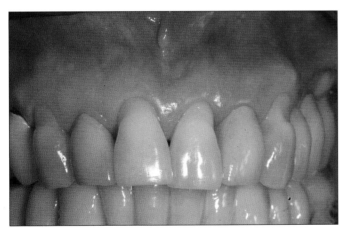

Figure 14.88. Another view of the completed case reveals the good aesthetic integration of the three-unit implant-supported maxillary left fixed partial denture. Keratinized gingiva is buccal to the last implant.

When grafting around an implant, it is advisable to surgically collect a slightly thicker layer of epithelialized connective tissue as compared with grafting around a natural tooth. It has been hypothesized that with an increased thickness of the connective tissue portion of the graft, its capillary system is better preserved (Holbrook & Ochsenbein 1983; Miller 1987). A faster activation of this more intact vascular network, in a thicker graft, may compensate for a reduction in the plasmic circulation originating from the peri-implant recipient bed (Sullivan & Atkins 1968; Miller 1987).

The combination of the absence of the periodontal ligament, the presence of a more cortical quality of the bone, and the reduced presence of vessels in the peri-implant soft tissues reduces the nourishment to the graft, which may necrotize and eventually slough off. To increase further the chances of graft survival, additional factors must be considered: the concordance between the dimension of the recipient site and the graft itself, an adequate hemostasis between the graft and its periosteal bed, and a tight adaptation between the graft and the underlying periosteum. The proper adaptation of the free gingival graft to the recipient area is provided, and maintained, by the suturing technique, which should ensure a light compression of the surgical area while stabilizing the graft in place (Smukler & Chaibi 1997).

PAPILLA REGENERATION TECHNIQUES

As discussed at the beginning of this chapter, there appears to be limitations to what is nowadays possible to achieve in terms of re-creation of lost papillary tissues (Tarnow et al. 2003). This is especially true for multiple implant rehabilitations. Several techniques have been designed (Salama et al. 1995; Adriaenssens et al. 1999; Palacci & Ericsson 2001; Tinti & Benfenati 2002; Smukler et al. 2003a & b) in the attempt to idealize the shape of the lost papilla surgically. Refer to this chapter's references for the description of sources on the different surgical procedures.

CONCLUSION

It is important to remember that, aside from the selected surgical approach for uncovering, the final presence of good papillae and gingival scallop surrounding the implant(s) depends on several other, previously mentioned factors. Consideration of these factors in the surgical approach is necessary to achieve a properly designed prosthetic restoration, which is of the utmost importance (Smukler et al. 2003a & b).

The carefully customized anatomical shape of the temporary prosthesis should start molding the surrounding peri-implant soft tissues as soon as possible. It is important to evaluate the degree of maturation of the soft tissue when exerting strategically located pressure to plot the peri-implant gingival profiles. A mature thick tissue can withstand higher degrees of pressure when compared with still-healing thin tissue, which could react to the push with a sudden undesirable recession.

Once the proper prosthetic sculpting of the gingiva has been achieved, the final restoration can be positioned. It is the responsibility of the surgeon to provide the prosthodontist with the right quality and quantity of hard and soft tissues to start the prosthetic molding process. Achieving the desired result is of utmost importance and depends on the continuous and harmonious interaction between the caregivers (i.e., the surgeon, prosthodontist, dental technician, and hygienist) and the patient.

At the conclusion of active treatment, a carefully designed individual maintenance program will ensure the long-term success of the procedure.

REFERENCES

Abrahamsson, I., Berglundh, T., & Lindhe, J. (1997) The mucosal barrier following abutment disconnection or reconnection: An experimental study in dogs. *Journal of Clinical Periodontology* 24, 568–572.

Abrahamsson, I., Zitzmann, N.U., Berglundh, T., Linder, E., Wennerberg, A., & Lindhe, J. (2002) The mucosal attachment to titanium implants with different surface characteristics: An experimental study in dogs. *Journal of Clinical Periodontology* 29, 448–455.

Abrams, L. (1980) Augmentation of the deformed residual edentulous ridge for fixed prosthesis. *Compendium of Continuing Education in Dentistry* 1, 205–214.

Adell, R., Lekholm, U., Rockler, B., & Brånemark, P.–I. (1981) A 15-year study of osseointegrated implants in the treatment of the edentulous jaw. *International Journal of Oral and Maxillofacial Surgery* 10, 387–416.

Adriaenssens, P., Hermans, M., Ingber, A., Prestipino, V., Daelemans, P., & Malevez, C. (1999) Palatal sliding strip flap: Soft tissue management to restore maxillary anterior esthetics at stage 2 surgery—A clinical report. *International Journal of Oral and Maxillofacial Surgery* 14, 30–36.

Alpert, A. (1994) A rationale for attached gingiva at the soft-tissue/implant interface: Esthetic and functional dictates. *Compendium of Continuing Education in Dentistry* 15, 356–366.

Apse, P., Zarb, G.A., Schmitt, A., & Lewis, D.W. (1991) The longitudinal effectiveness of osseointegrated dental implants. The Toronto Study: Peri-implant mucosal response. *International Journal of Periodontics Restorative Dentistry* 11, 94–111.

Astrand, P., Engquist, B., Dahlgren, S., Grondahl, K., Engquist, E., & Feldmann, H. (2004) Astra Tech and Brånemark system implants: A 5-year prospective study of marginal bone reactions. *Clinical Oral Implants Research* 15, 413–420.

Barone, R., Clauser, C., & Prato, G.P. (1999) Localized soft tissue ridge augmentation at phase 2 implant surgery: A case report. *International Journal of Periodontics Restorative Dentistry* 19, 141–145.

Becker, W., Ochsenbein, C., Tibbetts, L., & Becker, B.E. (1997) Alveolar bone anatomic profiles as measured from dry skulls: Clinical ramifications. *Journal of Clinical Periodontology* 24, 727–731.

Berglundh, T., & Lindhe, J. (1996) Dimension of the peri-implant mucosa: Biological width revisited. *Journal of Clinical Periodontology* 23, 971–973.

Berglundh, T., Lindhe, J., Ericsson, I., Marinello, C.P., Liljenberg, B., & Thomsen, P. (1991) The soft tissue barrier at implants and teeth. *Clinical Oral Implants Research* 2, 81–90.

Berglundh, T., Lindhe, J., Jonsson, K., & Ericsson, I. (1994) The topography of the vascular systems in the periodontal and peri-implant tissues in the dog. *Journal of Clinical Periodontology* 21, 189–193.

Bruno, J.F. (1994) Connective tissue graft technique assuring wide root coverage. *International Journal of Periodontics Restorative Dentistry* 14, 126–137.

Dharmar, S., Yoshida, K., Adachi, Y., Kishi, M., Okuda, K., & Sekine, H. (1994) Subgingival microbial flora associated with Brånemark implants. *International Journal of Periodontics Restorative Dentistry* 9, 314–318.

Dordick, B., Coslet, J.G., & Seibert, J.S. (1976) Clinical evaluation of free autogenous gingival grafts placed on alveolar bone. Part II. Coverage of nonpathologic dehiscences and fenestrations. *Journal of Periodontology* 47, 568–573.

Ericsson, I., Nilner, K., Klinge, B., & Glantz, P.O. (1996) Radiographical and histological characteristics of submerged and nonsubmerged titanium implants: An experimental study in the Labrador dog. *Clinical Oral Implants Research* 7, 20–26.

Friedmann, A., Strietzel, F.P., Maretzki, B., Pitaru, S., & Bernimoulin, J.P. (2002) Histological assessment of augmented jaw bone utilizing a new collagen barrier membrane compared to a standard barrier membrane to protect a granular bone substitute material. *Clinical Oral Implants Research* 13, 587–594.

Garber, D.A., & Belser, U.C. (1995) Restoration-driven implant placement with restoration-generated site development. *Compendium of Continuing Education in Dentistry* 16, 796, 798–802, 804.

Garber, D.A., Salama, M.A., & Salama, H. (2001) Immediate total tooth replacement. *Compendium of Continuing Education Dentistry* 22, 210–216, 218.

Gargiulo, A.W., Wentz, F.M., & Orban, B. (1961) Dimensions and relations of the dentogingival junction in humans. *Journal of Periodontology* 32, 261–267.

Goldman, H.M., & Cohen, D.W. (1980) *Periodontal Therapy*, 6th edition. St. Louis: C.V. Mosby, 670–677.

Grunder, U. (2000) Stability of the mucosal topography around single-tooth implants and adjacent teeth: One-year results. *International Journal of Periodontics and Restorative Dentistry* 20, 11–17.

Grunder, U., Gracis, S., & Capelli, M. (2005) Influence of the 3-D bone-to-implant relationship on esthetics. *International Journal of Periodontics and Restorative Dentistry* 25, 113–119.

Harris, R.J. (1994) The connective tissue with partial thickness double pedicle graft: The results of 100 consecutively treated defects. *Journal of Periodontology* 65, 448–461.

Hermann, J.S., Cochran, D.L., Nummikoski, P.V., & Buser, D. (1997) Crestal bone changes around titanium implants: A radiographic evaluation of unloaded nonsubmerged and submerged implants in the canine mandible. *Journal of Periodontology* 68, 1117–1130.

Hermann, J.S., Buser, D., Schenk, R.K., & Cochran, D.L. (2000) Crestal bone changes around titanium implants: A histometric evaluation of unloaded nonsubmerged and submerged implants in the canine mandible. *Journal of Periodontology* 71, 1412–1424.

Hermann, J.S., Buser, D., Schenk, R.K., Schoolfield, J.D., & Cochran, D.L. (2001) Biologic Width around one- and two-piece titanium implants. *Clinical Oral Implants Research* 12, 559–571.

Hertel, R.C., Blijdorp, P.A., Kalk, W., & Baker, D.L. (1994) Stage II surgical techniques in endosseous implantation. *International Journal of Oral Maxillofacial Implants* 9, 273–278.

Holbrook, T., & Ochsenbein, C. (1983) Complete coverage of the denuded root surface with a one-stage gingival graft. *International Journal of Periodontics Restorative Dentistry* 3(3), 8–27.

Holt, R.L., Rosenberg, M.M., Zinser, P.J., & Ganeles, J. (2002) A concept for a biologically derived, parabolic implant design. *International Journal of Periodontics Restorative Dentistry* 22, 473–481.

Hurzeler, M.B., & Weng, D. (1996) Peri-implant tissue management: Optimal timing for an aesthetic result. *Practical Periodontics and Aesthetic Dentistry* 8, 857–869; quiz, 869.

Israelson, H., & Plemons, J.M. (1993) Dental implants, regenerative techniques, and periodontal plastic surgery to restore maxillary anterior esthetics. *International Journal of Oral Maxillofacial and Implants* 8, 555–561.

Jovanovic, S.A., & Nevins, M. (1995) Bone formation utilizing titanium-reinforced barrier membranes. *International Journal of Periodontics and Restorative Dentistry* 15, 56–69.

Kois, J.C. (1996) The restorative-periodontal interface: Biological parameters. *Periodontology 2000* 11, 29–38.

Kon, S., Caffesse, R.G., Castelli, W.A., & Nasjleti, C.E. (1984) Vertical releasing incisions for flap design: Clinical and histological study in monkeys. *International Journal of Periodontics and Restorative Dentistry* 4, 48–57.

Landi, L., & Sabatucci, D. (2001) Plastic surgery at the time of membrane removal around mandibular endosseous implants: A modified technique for implant uncovering. *International Journal of Periodontics and Restorative Dentistry* 21, 280–287.

Lang, N.P., Wilson, T.G., & Corbet, E.F. (2000) Biological complications with dental implants: Their prevention, diagnosis, and treatment. *Clinical Oral Implants Research* 1, 146–155.

Langer, B., & Calagna L. (1980) The subepithelial connective tissue graft. *Journal of Prosthetic Dentistry* 44, 363–367.

Langer, B., & Langer, L. (1985) Subepithelial connective tissue graft technique for root coverage. *Journal of Periodontology* 56, 715–720.

Listgarten, M.A., Lang, N.P., Schroeder, H.E., & Schroeder, A. (1991) Periodontal tissues and their counterparts around endosseous implants. *Clinical Oral Implants Research* 2(3), 1–19.

Maynard, J.G., Jr., & Wilson, R.D. (1979) Physiologic dimensions of the periodontium significant to the restorative dentist. *Journal of Periodontology* 50, 170–174.

Miller, P.D., Jr. (1987) Root coverage with the free gingival graft: Factors associated with incomplete coverage. *Journal of Periodontology* 58, 674–681.

Moon, I.S., Berglundh, T., Abrahamsson, I., Linder, E., & Lindhe, J. (1999) The barrier between the keratinized mucosa and the dental implant: An experimental study in the dog. *Journal of Clinical Periodontology* 26, 658–663.

Mormann, W., & Ciancio, S.G. (1977) Blood supply of human gingiva following periodontal surgery: A fluorescein angiographic study. *Journal of Periodontology* 48, 681–692.

Moy, P.K., Weinlaender, M., & Kenney, E.B. (1989) Soft-tissue modifications of surgical techniques for placement and uncovering of osseointegrated implants. *Dental Clinics of North America* 33, 665–681.

Muller, H.P., & Eger, T. (2002) Masticatory mucosa and periodontal phenotype: A review. *International Journal of Periodontics and Restorative Dentistry* 22, 172–183.

Nelson, S.W. (1987) The subpedicle connective tissue graft: A bilaminar reconstructive procedure for the coverage of denuded root surfaces. *Journal of Periodontology* 58, 95–102.

Nemcovsky, C.E., Artzi, Z., & Moses, O. (1999) Rotated split palatal flap for soft tissue primary coverage over extraction sites with immediate implant placement: Description of the surgical procedure and clinical results. *Journal of Periodontology* 70, 926–934.

Nemcovsky, C.E., Moses, O., Artzi, Z., & Gelernter, I. (2000) Clinical coverage of dehiscence defects in immediate implant procedures: Three surgical modalities to achieve primary soft tissue closure. *International Journal of Oral and Maxillofacial Implants* 15, 843–852.

Nevins, M., & Mellonig, J.T. (1998) *Implant Therapy: Clinical Approaches and Evidence of Success.* Carol Stream, IL: Quintessence, 227.

Olsson, M., Lindhe, J., & Marinello, C.P. (1993) On the relationship between crown form and clinical features of the gingiva in adolescents. *Journal of Clinical Periodontology* 20, 570–577.

Palacci, P., & Ericsson, I. (2001) *Esthetic Implant Dentistry: Soft & Hard Tissue.* Carol Stream, IL: Quintessence.

Piattelli, A., Scarano, A., Piattelli, M., Bertolai, R., & Panzoni, E. (1997) Histologic aspects of the bone and soft tissues surrounding three titanium non-submerged plasma-sprayed implants retrieved at autopsy: A case report. *Journal of Periodontology* 68, 694–700.

Puchades-Roman, L., Palmer, R.M., Palmer, P.J., Howe, L.C., Ide, M., & Wilson, R.F. (2000) A clinical, radiographic, and microbiologic comparison of Astra Tech and Brånemark single tooth implants. *Clinical Implant Dentistry and Related Research* 2, 78–84.

Rosenquist, B. (1997) A comparison of various methods of soft tissue management following the immediate placement of implants into extraction sockets. *International Journal of Oral and Maxillofacial Implants* 12, 43–51.

Saadoun, A.P. (1997) The key to peri-implant esthetics: Hard- and soft-tissue management. *Dental Implantology Update* 8(6), 41–46.

Saadoun, A.P., & LeGall, M. (1992) Implant positioning for periodontal, functional, and aesthetic results. *Practical Periodontics and Aesthetic Dentistry* 4, 43–54.

Salama, H., Salama, M., Garber, D., & Adar, P. (1995) Developing optimal peri-implant papillae within the esthetic zone: Guided soft tissue augmentation. *Journal of Esthetic Dentistry* 7, 125–129.

Salama, H., Salama, M.A., Garber, D., & Adar, P. (1998) The interproximal height of bone: A guidepost to predictable aesthetic strategies and soft tissue contours in anterior tooth replacement. *Practical Periodontics and Aesthetic Dentistry* 10, 1131–1141.

Scharf, D.R., & Tarnow, D.P. (1992) Modified roll technique for localized alveolar ridge augmentation. *International Journal of Periodontics and Restorative Dentistry* 12, 415–425.

Schroeder, A., Van der Zypen, E., Stich, H., & Sutter, F. (1981) The reactions of bone, connective tissue, and epithelium to endosteal implants with titanium-sprayed surfaces. *Journal of Maxillofacial Surgery* 9, 15–25.

Sclar, A.J. (2003) *Soft Tissue and Esthetic Considerations in Implant Therapy.* Carol Stream, IL: Quintessence, 142–143.

Silverstein, L.H., Kurtzman, D., Garnick, J.J., Trager, P.S., & Waters, P.K. (1994) Connective tissue grafting for improved implant esthetics: Clinical technique. *Implant Dentistry* 3, 231–234.

Simion, M., Trisi, P., & Piattelli, A. (1994) Vertical ridge augmentation using a membrane technique associated with osseointegrated implants. *International Journal of Periodontics and Restorative Dentistry* 14, 496–511.

Smukler, H., & Chaibi, M. (1997) Periodontal and dental considerations in clinical crown extension: A rational basis for treatment. *International Journal of Periodontics and Restorative Dentistry* 17, 464–477.

Smukler, H., & Dreyer, C.J. (1969) Principal fibres of the periodontium. *Journal of Periodontal Research* 4, 19–25.

Smukler, H., Castellucci, F., & Capri, D. (2003a) The role of the implant housing in obtaining aesthetics: Generation of peri-implant gingivae and papillae. Part 1. *Practical Procedures and Aesthetic Dentistry* 15, 141–149.

Smukler, H., Castellucci, F., & Capri, D.T. (2003b) The role of the implant housing in obtaining aesthetics. Part 2. Customizing the peri-implant soft tissue. *Practical Procedures and Aesthetic Dentistry* 15, 487–490.

Staffileno, H., Levy, S., & Gargiulo, A. (1966) Histologic study of cellular mobilization and repair following a periosteal retention operation via split thickness mucogingival flap surgery. *Journal of Periodontology* 37, 117–131.

Sullivan, H.C., & Atkins, J.H. (1968) Free autogenous gingival grafts. 1. Principles of successful grafting. *Periodontics* 6, 5–13.

Tarnow, D.P., Magner, A.W., & Fletcher, P. (1992) The effect of the distance from the contact point to the crest of bone on the presence or absence of the interproximal dental papilla. *Journal of Periodontology* 63, 995–996.

Tarnow, D.P., Cho, S.C., & Wallace, S.S. (2000) The effect of inter-implant distance on the height of inter-implant bone crest. *Journal of Periodontology* 71, 546–549.

Tarnow, D., Elian, N., Fletcher, P., Froum, S., Magner, A., Cho, S.C., Salama, M., Salama, H., & Garber, D.A. (2003) Vertical distance from the crest of bone to the height of the interproximal papilla between adjacent implants. *Journal of Periodontology* 74, 1785–1788.

Tinti, C., & Benfenati, S.P. (2002) The ramp mattress suture: A new suturing technique combined with a surgical procedure to obtain papillae between implants in the buccal area. *International Journal of Periodontics and Restorative Dentistry* 22, 63–69.

Tinti, C., & Parma-Benfenati, S. (1995) Coronally positioned palatal sliding flap. *International Journal of Periodontics and Restorative Dentistry* 15, 298–310.

Triaca, A., Minoretti, R., Merli, M., & Merz, B. (2001) Periosteoplasty for soft tissue closure and augmentation in preprosthetic surgery: A surgical report. *International Journal of Oral and Maxillofacial Implants* 16, 851–856.

Vacek, J.S., Gher, M.E., Assad, D.A., Richardson, A.C., & Giambarresi, L.I. (1994) The dimensions of the human dentogingival junction. *International Journal of Periodontics and Restorative Dentistry* 14, 154–165.

Warrer, K., Buser, D., Lang, N.P., & Karring, T. (1995) Plaque-induced peri-implantitis in the presence or absence of keratinized mucosa: An experimental study in monkeys. *Clinical Oral Implants Research* 6, 131–138.

Weisgold, A.S., Arnoux, J.P., & Lu, J. (1997) Single-tooth anterior implant: A world of caution. Part I. *Journal of Esthetic Dentistry* 9, 225–233.

Wennstrom, J.L., Bengazi, F., & Lekholm, U. (1994) The influence of the masticatory mucosa on the peri-implant soft tissue condition. *Clinical Oral Implants Research* 5, 1–8.

Wöhrle, P.S. (2003) Nobel Perfect esthetic scalloped implant: Rationale for a new design. *Clinical Implant Dentistry and Related Research* 5, 64–73.

Zitzmann, N.U., Naef, R., & Scharer, P. (1997) Resorbable versus non-resorbable membranes in combination with Bio-Oss for guided bone regeneration. *International Journal of Oral and Maxillofacial Implants* 12, 844–852.

Chapter 15: Improving Patients' Smiles: Aesthetic Crown-Lengthening Procedure

Serge Dibart

HISTORY

There are two aspects to the crown lengthening procedure: aesthetic and functional. In both cases, the surgical procedure is aimed at reestablishing the biological width apically while exposing more tooth structure. The biological width is defined as the sum of the junctional epithelium and supracrestal connective tissue attachment (Cohen 1962).

Gargiulo et al. (1961), who measured the human dentogingival junction, found that the average space occupied by the sum of the junctional epithelium and the supracrestal connective tissue fibers is 2.04 mm. Violation of that space by restorations impinging on the biological width has been associated with gingival inflammation, discomfort, gingival recession, alveolar bone loss, pocket formation, and the like (Parma-Benfenati et al. 1985; Tarnow et al. 1986; Tal et al. 1989).

To have a harmonious and successful long-term restoration, Ingber et al. (1977) advocated 3 mm of sound supracrestal tooth structure between bone and prosthetic margins, which allows for the reformation of the biological width plus sulcus depth. This can be achieved surgically (crown lengthening) or orthodontically (forced eruption) or by a combination of both (Ingber 1976; Pontoriero et al. 1987; De Waal and Castellucci 1994).

INDICATIONS

- To improve the gummy smile of a patient with a high smile line

- To rehabilitate dentition that is compromised by the presence of extensive caries, short clinical crowns, traumatic injuries, or severe parafunctional habits

- To restore gingival health when the biological width has been violated by a prosthetic restoration that is too close to the alveolar bone crest

Crown lengthening can be limited to the soft tissues when there is enough gingiva coronal to the alveolar bone, allowing for surgical modification of the gingival margins without the need for osseous recontouring (that is, pseudopockets in cases of gingival hyperplasia). An external or internal bevel gingivectomy (gingivoplasty) is the procedure of choice in these cases.

The biological width has not been compromised, and, as a result, the soft tissue pocket is eliminated and the teeth exposed without the need for osseous resection. Unfortunately, the majority of cases will involve bone recontouring as well as gingival resection to accommodate aesthetics and function. This is a more delicate procedure that requires exposing root surface, positioning gingival margins at the desired height, and apically reestablishing the biological width.

The crown-lengthening procedure enables restorative dentists to develop an adequate zone for crown retention without extending the crown margins deep into periodontal tissues. After the procedure, it is customary to wait 6–8 weeks before cementing the final restoration. In the aesthetic zone, a waiting period of at least 6 months is recommended before final impression (Pontoriero & Carnevale 2001). This reduces the chances of gingival recession following prosthetic crown insertion, specifically if there is a thin biotype.

A FEW WORDS ABOUT AESTHETICS

As the saying goes, "Beauty is in the eye of the beholder." Oral aesthetics is part art and part science. The enhancement of a person's smile culminates in the individualization of the general rules governing dental aesthetics for that person. Every patient is different, and yet a nice smile is the result of an orderly combination of several components. Knowing the general guidelines that make a smile appealing and tailoring them to an individual patient gives that smile uniqueness.

The aesthetic zone has been defined as the area encompassed by the upper and lower lips (Saadoun & LeGall 1998). It is the harmonious relationship among the dentition (premolar to premolar), the periodontium (gingival line), and the lips that will make or break a smile.

In 1984, Tjan et al., after observing several hundred dental and hygiene students, defined a standard of normalcy in an aesthetic smile (Figs. 15.1 & 15.2).

ARMAMENTARIUM

This includes the basic kit plus crown-lengthening burrs and bone chisels.

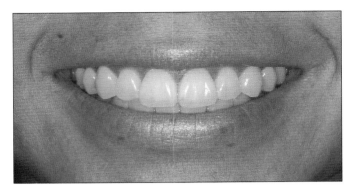

Figure 15.1. A pleasant smile line reveals 75%–100% of the maxillary anterior teeth and the interproximal gingiva only (68.94% of the subjects). The gingival margins of the central incisors and canines are located horizontally at the same level, whereas the gingival margins of the laterals are 2 mm below. The maxillary incisal curve is parallel with the lower lip (84.8% of the subjects). From Tjan et al. (1984).

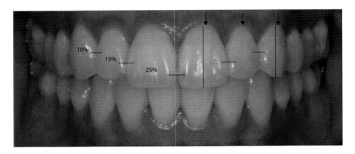

Figure 15.2. The position of the anterior contact point progressing from incisal to cervical and from central incisors to canines (*horizontal lines*). The location of the gingival zenith (*black arrows*), the most apical point of the gingival tissue, referencing the tooth axis, is distal on the maxillary central incisors and canines, and coincidental on lateral incisors (Rufenacht 2000). The *golden percentage* (25%, 15%, and 10%) is considered a starting point in designing the relative width of teeth in a beautiful smile. With all of these width ratios added together, the total canine-to-canine width becomes the *golden percentage* (Snow 1999).

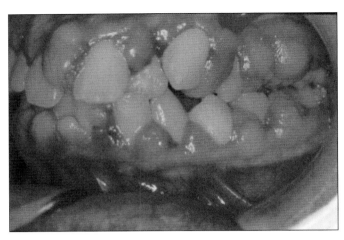

Figure 15.3. Gingival hyperplasia secondary to the daily use of Dilantin (phenytoin). This excessive tissue affects patients' dental aesthetics and function.

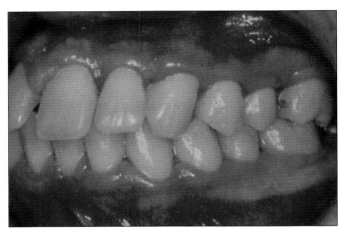

Figure 15.4. The mouth of a patient after minor orthodontic treatment and full-mouth external bevel gingivectomy. Hyperplastic gingival tissue has been surgically eliminated and the teeth exposed to the oral environment. As there is no need for osseous recontouring, the biological width is undisturbed.

SOFT TISSUE CROWN LENGTHENING

Soft tissue crown lengthening is best accomplished with an external or internal bevel gingivectomy. The alveolar bone is left intact, the depth of the soft tissue pocket is marked with a probe (bleeding points) and a gingivectomy knife, Kirkland (Hu-Friedy, Chicago, IL, USA) or Orban (Hu-Friedy) (in case of external bevel gingivectomy), or a no. 15 blade (internal bevel gingivectomy) is used to eliminate that excess gingival (Figs. 15.3 and 15.4).

HARD TISSUE CROWN LENGTHENING

The optimal gingival line (margins) is determined after careful evaluation of the diagnostic waxup. A surgical guide is prepared from the waxup model that will help the surgeon re-create the ideal gingival line in the mouth. Using a no. 15 blade as a pencil, the surgeon outlines the incision and, following the surgical guide, keeps the blade at an angle to create a coronal internal bevel.

The full-thickness flap is then reflected, the secondary flap discarded, and the bone exposed. Using burrs or bone chisels, the alveolar bone is recontoured to create a 3-mm space between the bone and the anticipated new margins. The flaps are sutured back in place and the area left to heal for about 3 weeks before repreparing the teeth (supragingivally) and relining the temporaries. A waiting period of about 6 months, in temporaries, is recommended in the aesthetic zone before final preparation and restoration (Figs. 15.5–15.14).

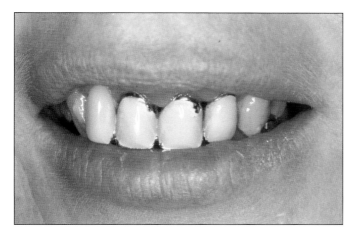

Figure 15.5. The mouth of a 42-year-old woman unhappy with her smile. Her lip line shows maxillary gingiva, iatrogenic dentistry, and erroneous gingival margin positions.

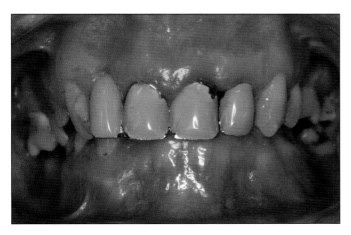

Figure 15.6. Intraoral photography shows a poorly designed prosthesis, severe overbite, faulty crown margins, and severely decayed teeth.

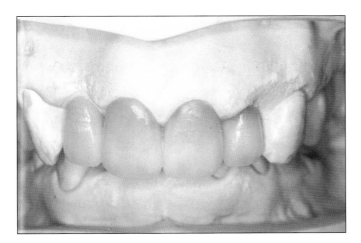

Figure 15.7. Diagnostic waxup from which a surgical guide will be created.

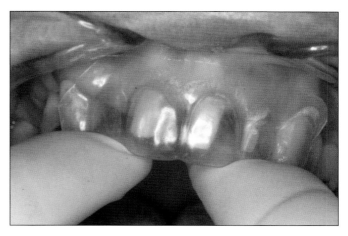

Figure 15.8. The provisional restorations are removed, and the surgical guide created from the waxup is inserted. This guides the surgeon to position the new gingival margins to the desired levels. The surgical incision follows the surgical guide closely to give the restorative dentist the precise amount of tooth structure needed to create a new gingival architecture.

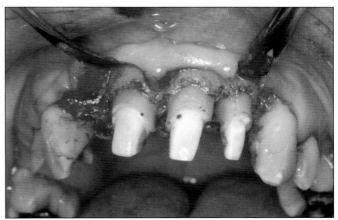

Figure 15.9. The full-thickness flap is elevated, and the osseous recontouring is done to expose the new tooth structure that will receive the new prosthetic margins. A 3-mm space between the bone crest and the planned new prosthetic margins is imperative for successful restora-

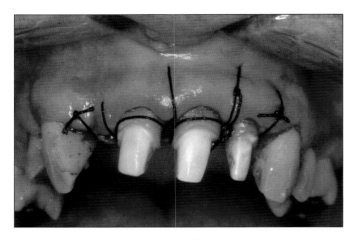

Figure 15.10. The flaps are secured with a continuous sling and vertical mattress suture.

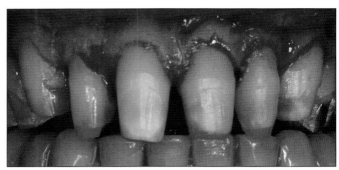

Figure 15.13. The surgical crown-lengthening procedure performed with removal of hard and soft tissues.

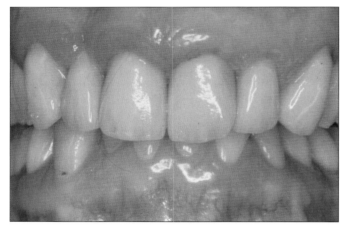

Figure 15.11. The final prosthesis is inserted 1 year later. The teeth have been customized to fit the patient's morphogenetic type.

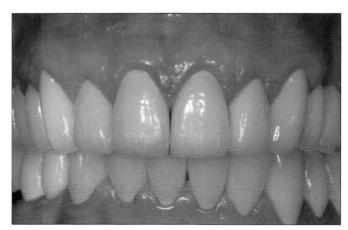

Figure 15.14. A patient's mouth rehabilitated aesthetically and functionally with individual porcelain fused to metal crowns.

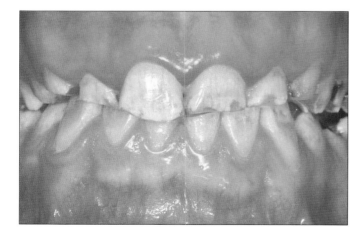

Figure 15.12. The mouth of a patient who has amelogenesis imperfecta. Extensive decay and short clinical crowns make it difficult for proper rehabilitation without crown lengthening.

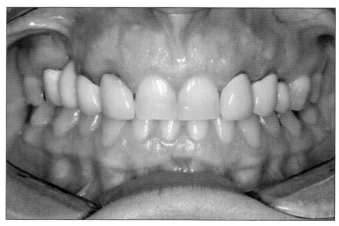

Figure 15.15. The mouth of a 40-year-old woman unhappy with her smile. She seeks help to improve her appearance and boost her self-confidence.

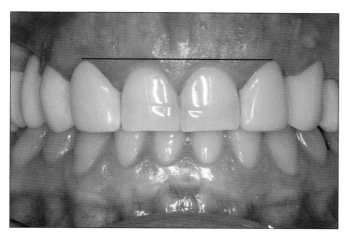

Figure 15.16. The mouth of the same patient after caries control and temporization. The condition has somewhat improved but notice the erroneous position of the gingival margins of teeth 8 and 9. They should be situated above the gingival margins of the lateral incisors.

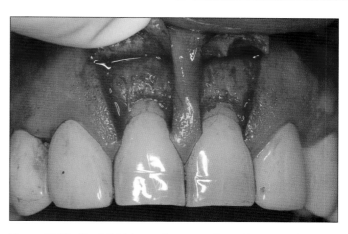

Figure 15.19. The full-thickness flaps are reflected just enough to expose crestal bone. The interdental papilla is left alone; this enhances a positive aesthetic outcome.

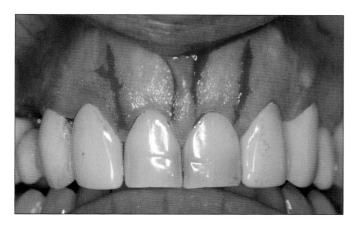

,Figure 15.17. Two short vertical buccal incisions at the line angles of teeth 8 and 9 are made with a microblade leaving papillae and frenum intact. The mesial incisions are hidden in the labial frenum; this allows for invisible scarring.

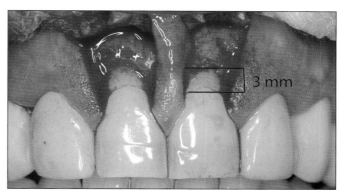

Figure 15.20. Crestal bone is removed with a chisel or a burr to have 3 mm of space between the anticipated prosthetic margins and the alveolar bone.

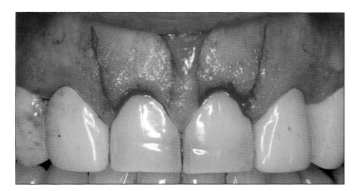

Figure 15.18. A submarginal incision mimicking the final gingival margin levels of teeth 8 and 9 will help connect the two verticals.

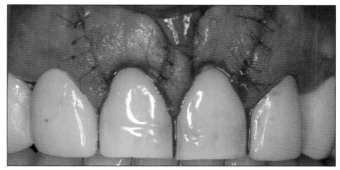

Figure 15.21. The flaps are sutured back in place with resorbable 7-0 microsutures. The number and position of the microsutures enable a close adaptation of the flaps and subsequent rapid healing.

MICROSURGICAL CROWN LENGTHENING

In the areas of high aesthetic demand, where papilla and soft tissue conservation is of paramount importance, the use of a microsurgical technique is recommended. There will be smaller incisions, which will not involve the papillae.

Flap reflection is minimal, and the sutures enable a very close adaptation of the flaps. This, in turn, results in minimal inflammation, scarring, and patient discomfort. Because of the minimally invasive nature of the procedures and the superior wound adaptation, quick healing and enhanced aesthetics are to be expected (Figs. 15.15–15.23)

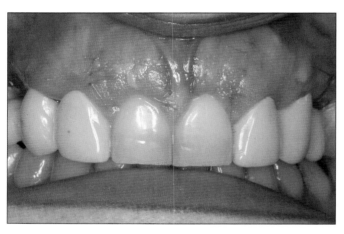

Figure 15.22. The mouth of the patient 1 week later. Notice the quality of the wound healing.

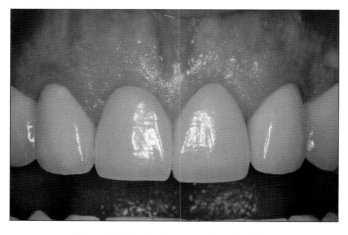

Figure 15.23. Final veneers 4 months later.

REFERENCES

Cohen, D.W. (1962) Periodontal preparation of the mouth for restorative dentistry. Presented at the Walter Reed Army Medical Center, Washington, DC, 3 June 1962.

De Waal, H., & Castellucci, G. (1994) The importance of restorative margin placement to the biologic width and periodontal health. Part II. *International Journal of Periodontics and Restorative Dentistry* 14, 70–83.

Gargiulo, A.W., Wentz, F.M., & Orban, B. (1961) Dimensions and relations of the dentogingival junction in humans. *Journal of Periodontology* 32, 261–267.

Ingber, J.S. (1976) Forced eruption. Part II. A method of treating nonrestorable teeth: Periodontal and restorative considerations. *Journal of Periodontology* 47, 203–213.

Ingber, F.J.S., Rose, L.F., & Coslet, J.G. (1977) The biologic width: A concept in periodontics and restorative dentistry. *Alpha Omegan* 10, 62–65.

Parma-Benfenati, S., Fugazzotto, P.A., & Ruben, M.P. (1985) The effect of restorative margins on the post-surgical development and nature of the periodontium. Part I. *International Journal of Periodontics and Restorative Dentistry* 5(6), 30–51.

Pontoriero, R., & Carnevale, G. (2001) Surgical crown lengthening: A 12-month clinical wound healing study. *Journal of Periodontology* 72, 841–848.

Pontoriero, R., Celenza, F., Jr., Ricci, G., & Carnevale, M. (1987) Rapid extrusion with fiber resection: A combined orthodontic-periodontic treatment modality. *International Journal of Periodontics and Restorative Dentistry* 5, 30–43.

Rufenacht, C.R. (2000) *Principles of Esthetic Integration.* London: Quintessence, 13–36.

Saadoun, A.P., & LeGall, M.G. (1998) Periodontal implications in implant treatment planning for aesthetic results. *Practical Periodontics and Aesthetic Dentistry* 10, 655–664.

Snow, S.R. (1999) Esthetic smile analysis of maxillary anterior tooth width: The golden percentage. *Journal of Esthetic Dentistry* 11, 177–184.

Tal, H., Soldinger, M., Dreiangel, A., & Pitaru, S. (1989) Periodontal response to long-term abuse of the gingival attachment by supracrestal amalgam restorations. *Journal of Clinical Periodontology* 16, 654–689.

Tarnow, D., Sthal, S.S., Magner, A., & Zamzok, J. (1986) Human gingival attachment responses to subgingival crown placement–marginal remodeling. *Journal of Clinical Periodontology* 13, 563–569.

Tjan, A.H., Miller, G.D., & The, J.G. (1984) Some esthetic factors in a smile. *Journal of Prosthetic Dentistry* 51, 24–28.

Chapter 16: Selection Criteria

Serge Dibart and Mamdouh Karima

The proper selection of the numerous techniques must be based on the predictability of success that, in turn, is based on the following criteria discussed in this chapter.

PLAQUE-FREE AND CALCULUS-FREE ENVIRONMENT

Periodontal plastic surgical procedures should be performed in a plaque-free and inflammation-free environment to enable firm gingival tissue management. When the tissue is inflamed and edematous, precise incision lines and flap reflection cannot be achieved. The patient's teeth must undergo careful and thorough scaling, root planning, and meticulous plaque control before any surgical procedure.

AESTHETIC DEMAND

Short-term clinical studies show that the connective tissue graft results in superior root coverage compared with the epithelialized free soft tissue graft. In addition, the color match of the grafted area to the adjacent gingiva is aesthetically more favorable with the connective tissue graft than with an epithelialized free graft.

ADEQUATE BLOOD SUPPLY

Maximum blood supply to the donor tissue is essential. Gingival augmentation apical to the area of recession benefits from a better blood supply than does coronal augmentation, because the recipient bed is entirely vascular (periosteum). Root-coverage procedures are a challenge because a portion of the bed is avascular (the portion of the root to be covered). Therefore, if aesthetics is not a factor, gingival augmentation apical to the recession may have a more predictable outcome.

A pedicle-displaced flap has a better blood supply than a free graft (since the base of the flap is intact in the former). Therefore, in root coverage, if the anatomy is favorable, the use of a pedicle flap or any of its variants may be the best procedure.

The pouch and tunnel techniques use a split flap for a subepithelial connective tissue graft, with the connective tissue sandwiched in between the flap. This flap design maximizes the blood supply to the donor tissue. If large areas require root coverage, these sandwich-type recipient sites provide the best flap design for blood supply.

ANATOMY OF THE RECIPIENT AND DONOR SITES

The anatomy of the recipient and donor sites is an important consideration in selecting the proper technique. The presence or absence of vestibular depth is an essential anatomical criterion at the recipient site for gingival augmentation. If gingival augmentation is indicated apical to the area of recession, there must be adequate vestibular depth apical to the recessed gingival margin to provide space for either a free or pedicle graft.

Only a free graft can accomplish vestibular depth apical to the recession. Use mucogingival techniques, such as free gingival grafts and free connective tissue grafts, to create vestibular depth and widen the zone of attached gingiva. Other techniques require the presence of the vestibule before the surgery. These procedures include pedicle grafts (lateral and coronal), subepithelial connective tissue grafts, and pouch and tunnel procedures.

DONOR TISSUE AVAILABILITY

Pedicle displacement of tissue necessitates the creation of an adjacent donor site presenting the appropriate gingival thickness and width. Palatal tissue thickness is necessary for the connective tissue donor autograft. Gingival thickness is also required at the recipient site for techniques using a split-thickness, sandwich-type flap, or pouch and tunnel techniques.

GRAFT STABILITY

Good anastomosis of the blood vessels from the grafted donor tissue to the recipient site requires a stable environment. This necessitates sutures that stabilize the donor tissue firmly against the recipient site. The goal is maximum stability with the least number of sutures.

TRAUMA

Like all surgical procedures, periodontal plastic surgery is based on the meticulous, delicate, and precise management of the oral tissue. Unnecessary tissue trauma caused by poor incisions, flap perforations, tears, or traumatic and excessive placement of sutures can lead to tissue necrosis. The selection of proper instruments, needles, and sutures is necessary to minimize tissue trauma. The use of sharp, contoured blades, smaller-diameter needles, and resorbable, monofilament sutures is important in achieving atraumatic surgery (Table 16.1).

TABLE 16.1. Treatment options for various clinical conditions

Existing condition	Proposed treatment
Lack of attached gingiva (≤1 mm). No recession. Lack of vestibular depth.	**Free gingival autograft**
Gingival recession (need for root coverage). Miller's (1985) class I and II.[a]	**Connective tissue graft** 3.3- to 5.9-mm recessions. Average percentage of root coverage, 91%. **Coronally advanced flap** 2.2- to 4.1-mm recession. Average percentage of root coverage, 83%. **Guided tissue regeneration** 4.6- to 6.3-mm recession. Average percentage of root coverage, 74%. **Free gingival autograft** 2.1- to 5.1-mm recessions. Average percentage of root coverage, 72%. **Rotational flaps** 3- to 5-mm recession. Average percentage of root coverage, 64%. **Two-stage procedure** Average percentage of root coverage, 63%.
Gingival recession. Miller's (1985) class III and IV.	**Incomplete root coverage** irrespective of the technique used.
High insertion of labial maxillary or mandibular frenum, frenum pull, recession.	**Frenectomy** for orthodontic treatment **Frenectomy** with or without free gingival autograft
Ridge deformities: Horizontal deficit, moderate 3- to 6-mm defect.[b]	**Fixed partial denture restoration planned** Soft tissue grafting (free gingival, connective tissue, Alloderm[c] grafts). **Implant supported prosthesis planned** Hard tissue grafting (GBR,[d] ERE[e]).
Ridge deformities: Horizontal and vertical deficits, severe defects ≥ 4 mm.[b]	**Fixed partial denture restoration planned** Soft tissue grafting (free gingival, connective tissue, AlloDerm[c] grafts). **Implant-supported prosthesis planned** Hard tissue grafting (GBR[d]), distraction osteogenesis. **Combination of soft and hard tissue grafting**
Extensive caries, short clinical crowns, traumatic injuries, or severe parafunctional habits. Compromised biological width.	**Crown-lengthening procedure** with resective osseous surgery
High smile line showing excessive amounts of gingiva resulting in patient's discontent with facial appearance. Altered passive eruption	
Excessive gingival tissue covering erupted dentition (gingival hyperplasia, hypertrophy, pseudo-gingival pockets).	**Soft tissue resective surgery** (internal/external bevel gingivectomy, gingivoplasty)

[a]Adapted from Wennstrom (1996).
[b]Adapted from Pini-Prato et al. (2004).
[c]Acellular dermal matrix Allograft.
[d]GBR, guided bone regeneration.
[e]ERE, edentulous ridge expansion.

REFERENCES

Miller, P.D., Jr. (1985) A classification of marginal tissue recession. *International Journal of Periodontics and Restorative Dentistry* 5:8–13.

Pini-Prato, G.P., Cairo, F., Tinti, C., Cortellini, P., Muzzi, L., & Mancini, E.A. (2004) Prevention of alveolar ridge deformities and reconstruction of lost anatomy: A review of surgical approaches. *International Journal of Periodontics and Restorative Dentistry* 24, 435–445.

Wennstrom, J.L. (1996) Mucogingival therapy. *Annals of Periodontology* 1, 671–701.

Index